Janet Todd, novelist (*A Man of Genius*, 2016) and internationally renowned scholar, was until recently President of Lucy Cavendish College, Cambridge. Born in Wales, she grew up in Ceylon, Bermuda, and the UK. She was a Professor of English at Rutgers University, NJ, and at the Universities of East Anglia, Glasgow and Aberdeen. She has also worked as an academic in Ghana, Puerto Rico, and India. An expert on women's writing and feminism and co-founder of the journal *Women's Writing*, she has published biographies and critical work on many authors, including Jane Austen, the Shelley Circle, Mary Wollstonecraft, and Aphra Behn. Now an Honorary Fellow of Newnham College, she lives in Cambridge and Venice. She is completing her third novel, *Don't You Know There's a War On?*

'Gripping, original, with abundant thrills, spills and revelations'

The Lady

'A haunting, sophisticated story' *Sunday Times*

'A real knack for language with some jaw-droppingly luscious dialogue. I can see the author's pedigree in the story, style and substance of the book: think *The Elegance of the Hedgehog*'

Geoffrey Jennings, Rainy Day Books

'Janet Todd is one of the foremost feminist literary historians writing in this country. She has devoted her literary career to recovering the lives and works of women writers overlooked and disparaged by generations of male literary scholars'

Lisa Jardine, *Independent on Sunday*

'Janet Todd guides us with unfailing buoyancy and a wit all her own. [Behn] is now wondrously resurrected'

Michael Foot, *Evening Standard*

'Thorough and stimulating. A fascinating study'

Maureen Duffy, *Literary Review*

'Janet Todd, a feminist scholar, has done a great deal of ground-breaking scholarship on women writers of the 'long eighteenth century'. [Her work] reads quickly and lightly. Even Todd's throw-away lines are steeped in learning and observation. Todd has documented so ably the daring attempt of a woman to write, both for her daily bread and for immortal fame'

Ruth Perry, *Women's Review of Books*

Radiation Diaries

Cancer, Memory and Fragments
of a Life in Words

JANET TODD

Fentum
Press

Fentum Press, London

Sold and distributed by Global Book Sales/Macmillan Distribution
and in North America by Consortium Book Sales and Distribution, Inc.,
part of the Ingram Content Group.

A CIP catalogue record for this book is available from the British Library

ISBN (paperback) 978-1-909572-17-1

Typeset by Palimpsest Book Production Limited, Falkirk,
Stirlingshire, Scotland

Printed and bound in Great Britain by
CPI Group (UK) Ltd, Croydon CRO 4YY

Radiation Diaries

It's near midwinter. I face over a month of whole pelvic radiotherapy. Being a wordy person, I need a verbal sedative: I resolve on a diary. The subject will be Life in Hospital-land.

Pro: a diary should prevent excessive talking of symptoms. As the president of a Cambridge college, I might embarrass colleagues who'd be too polite to protest. Writing should deliver a little detachment?

Con: a diary will be indecorous and excremental. See Web descriptions of Side- and After-Effects.

'The fox knows many things, the hedgehog only one.' This enigmatic saying is often interpreted as the hedgehog knows how to escape.

Rolling into a ball and displaying prickles seems to me a good metaphor for fear.

7 December, Wednesday

Around 4 a.m. my panicky Web-searching focuses on percentages of recovery from 3 cancers – strictly 2 cancers and a vault recurrence, but a little hyperbole is justified: treatment will be 'radical', serious, no half-and-half affair.

Sometimes the whole control group is dead after a year or so.

I think. A lifetime of reading and teaching reading and now I sit skimming words, unsure what I've seen.

Back to bed. I burrow under the duvet and beg the bladder for a truce. It refuses. As if it knows.

The first cancer, 2 years ago, was bladder – it weathered its chemo. Then came endometrial – and now a vaginal recurrence, demanding this brutal 'radical' treatment. Along with other organs down there, the chastened bladder will feel the fire. No wonder it's terrified and shivering.

Up again in under 10 minutes.

Must be on the road by 7.20 with kind D, whose healthy mornings – it was supposed to be his research leave – will be ruled by this, caught in another person's ordeal.

I'm too worried to drive. I visualise the grim concrete car park with me scraping its sharp pillars against the car's soft metal. The idea of the ageing car makes me almost teary. 'Aw shucks,' as Goofy used to say. Dead I suppose by now.

I hate but lean into the uncommon dependence.

D will drive deftly and slowly and we'll always arrive early.

Should I have breakfast? Brown toast and an orange too much? A banana? I so want to do the right thing.

I put on my new hospital kit: baggy red skirt from Laura Ashley to keep parts aired, no more sleek Viyella trousers from Jaeger; long socks from M&S to avoid pantyhose; waist-high cotton knickers, no synthetic briefs.

It's pitch dark as we leave. The car's clammy. We're silent. No sign of dawn, cold, wintry.

'Not my funeral,' I say.

A little deaf, D doesn't hear.

'What in me is dark illumine,' I mutter. This time D catches the sound and the reference. Not seeing the relevance of *Paradise Lost*. Me neither.

Switch on the sun, please.

In my solitary mid-teens, I filled a 5-year diary, not with my life, but with worthy quotations from Colin Wilson's *The Outsider* and masters like Thomas Mann or Aldous Huxley, who threw out their phrases world-wearily as partial truths. In Polonius style. 'This above all: to thine own self be true.' Sounds good till you unpack it, which I didn't then. 'Oh may I join the choir invisible' – recited at the Baptist social I assumed it implied dying to become a cherub trilling sweet notes: less jolly when I learnt it demanded 'daring rectitude'.

Since abandoning my snippets, I haven't looked in books for guidance. Just pleasure, exhilarating sometimes, consoling at others – like a solitary walk by the sea. I'm not finding much help from English Literature just now. Not even John Milton. Indeed, though useful in times of numbness, EngLit has never much served during the 'tumults and agitations of life'.

Nonetheless it sticks (some of it). 'Above the waste allotments the dawn halts' – see that aching word 'halts'. I've not thought of Dylan Thomas much in years – I suspect he's out of vogue – but he's back with me today.

Little on the road. Ample, tree-filled side-streets near the hospital, doctors' homes close to private schools?

We park in the damp multi-storey car park. A space on the first floor; must be too early for regular visitors. Step out into the murk, a Scandi-noir crime setting.

We walk down scruffy steps into the open air by the motorbike park, then cross to the main hospital. Nearby, a few evergreens look lank and ugly in the artificial yellowy light. Inside, a coloured mobile hangs motionless from a high ceiling. Stuck? Everything too sharply lit. Floor sticky. Or my shoe soles? Few people around. The coffee stall closed.

We lose our way.

I try to recall the cheerful artwork designed to guide us along tangling corridors and round clinics. Ariadne's thread for Theseus in her father's labyrinth, bound for the monster he's come to kill. Ovid found the girl forsaken and exposed on Naxos, imagining the miseries to come.

'Many different versions,' remarks D (who read Classics) when I mention the parallel. I raise an eyebrow, as usual.

We still can't remember the paintings.

Eventually we arrive, down the corridor with no natural light. 2 couples already in the waiting area. Silent. Is the man or woman growing a cancer? You can't ask. The men look grey and drink ice-cold water in thin paper cups.

Nobody tells me to do this. But I do it, ignoring gender, as we've learnt to do. Struggling to swallow, I worry. Will I be able to hold the water in my unruly bladder? How long will the treatment be? Will the great beam squash and squelch it?

Why didn't I study the process, the technicalities of treatment? Wasting time on percentages of death in the night.

The machine room is cold; it needs to be kept like this – or what? Will the monster throw a tantrum, stop? No 'decent drapery', no soft, pastel-blue hospital things. Just the hard, black top of the hard bed.

I pull off the red-tent Laura Ashley skirt to reveal my new purple tattoo marks required for the beam. (There forever – but 'forever' no longer seems so long.) Parts have been kept cool.

I try not to shiver.

2 young women attend the machine. Pleasant, efficient. I call them 'girls' to myself, regressing from decades of feminism – which, I see, hasn't been transformative.

3 of us here. 3 'women and a goose make a market.' Why this jingle in my head? A thin sandbag against thought? Why not something higher toned?

A boy band pulsates. If I don't have tinnitus now, I soon will.

I ask who chooses this music.

'Sometimes patients, sometimes us.'

The girls pull down my new baggy pants. They prod and pull the flesh, manoeuvring me into maximum pain. Tailbone presses into hard metal. Is it metal? No, carbon fibre. Hard as nails anyway. Ratchet up the bed.

They exit swiftly together, the green light carrying words I can't see turns red. I'm alone splayed out for the machine. No goose, no market. A woman alone. Corpse yoga pose without Lycra blue bottoms.

I haven't lain so rudely since a hectic bout of malaria in Ghana and I was discovered – and covered – by a gallant Fanti (Ghana being the politest society in all the world) 50 years back.

The hard surface is cold, cool air wafts round it. I expect a beam but there's only the ghostly green laser seeking purple marks.

I'm too short-sighted to notice much – I was told I had a lazy eye, then both eyes grew 'lazy'.

Spectacles have moved up my nose, I look under them. The red words form a fiery blur.

However, I do see close by a scrawny, flabby torso – maybe, like wood, it might be improved by arty distressing. Unpainted toenails reproach me: if I had proper *joie de vivre*, I'd have coloured them purple, or better fuchsia. Still, Old Body, we've come a long way together and taken some battering. Let's try to 'buck up'. No point in being enemies.

My feet are blocks of ice.

The green beam isn't the important part. It's what comes out of the machine, invisibly. The machine is a hammer, an arm without a body. There's a box one end, a round shape with a square eye on the other, above it 2 slit eyebrows of lit-up wires. Darkness beyond. The square eye matters, the box is its moon that rises when it sets, passing round and under your backside. The eye goes behind too, right round. I didn't expect that. (This isn't the place for anthropomorphism, I rebuke myself, but go on looking into the 'eye'.)

When the box is up, I stare into the machine's big dark squareness, my impotent eyes wide open, then quickly blink. I'm in Poe's Pit and Pendulum with Father Time's deep swinging sickle. I try not to breathe in case I move and upset the process: no French army nearby to ride to the rescue. The pain in my tailbone swirls up my back to my shoulders. Perhaps on later days I'll close my eyes. The boy band plays on. The bright overhead light has dimmed a little – or am I dying? The machine – its (his?) name is LA8 – hisses and peeps and shifts along like an old steam train on a branch line.

I'm lost without words. Nothing to read. *I have nothing to read.* I feel an addict's painful withdrawal. What's left of me if I'm not reading, talking or writing?

Old (almost repressed) memories swirl up. The long black socks echo those darned knee-highs, topped by navy-blue bloomers under a green gymslip.

I'm sitting alone on the platform at Crewe on my way to school – very still like now, struggling to breathe in the foul, black-speckled steam-train air, trying to take up less space, feeling the bristle of socks against the hairs on my legs. The fog is deep. A National Service-man comes by in his khaki uniform. Tries to talk to me, offers a cigarette. I'm 13 and bewildered, but want to be amiable. The tussle keeps me mum. He slouches off into the fog whistling 'Mona Lisa'. Another man, older, with a British Rail cap, comes by and says there won't be a train tonight and where was I bound anyhow? I say the Welsh name. He can't understand. I mangle it in English. He thinks me simple. I clutch my leather bag tightly. When he's gone I eat my thin sandwich, a mush of white bread and sugar in grease-proof paper.

Did the train ever come? It must have, for there were more years to get through in Dotheboys Hall.

Much later I studied Romantic lives, 1816, the summer without the sun when crops failed and people grew gloomy and gothic, inventing monsters and vampires. I thought of my 4 years in that school as such a sun-less time. More metaphoric than literal of course – though in truth there were plenty of sombre, cloud-covered days, allowing for much technicolour self-pity.

Usually I was there for half-term holidays, it being too difficult to get to my aunt in Mid-Wales by train or bus. But, for one, I was invited out by a gentle, withdrawn girl from the B class. After our glorious translation to Bermuda when I was 6, I knew Aunty's cold, damp Welsh house was no palace, but, until this visit to South Wales, I'd not seen urban poverty. The girl was a charity pupil; her small shabby home part of a terrace backing on to a slag heap that almost pushed against its back door. At the dark kitchen table sat a silent, depressed father, alcoholic I assume now, though I noticed nothing then, the smell of fat and soot overpowering any hint of beer or rum. He'd lost wife and son in an accident. He wished the girl, not the boy, had died.

The visit dented my epic self-pity. But soon it was energising me again. A common punishment was learning 20 lines of *Paradise Lost* Book I – soon my 'answering back' and unintentional bolshie ways landed me at Satan waging eternal, irreconcilable war by 'force or guile'.

My first session ends, the young girls return. A little impatient. Old hands know the ritual. I take too long pulling up knickers, putting on boots and skirt. I ask too many questions, thinking to be agreeable. The next man enters and jokes easily with them about their evening out.

I've been holding my breath too long under the machine. I gulp. It's over.

On the way home in the car, I think of Father and feel ashamed.

Way over 90 he went through this. Or worse, radiotherapy to the head, needing the face to be masked. Each day he travelled in the little hospital bus there and back by himself. Sometimes the trip was interminable, he said, taking in every housing estate and village; sometimes he held his aching head in both hands. Once the bus passed close to his flat, but couldn't deviate from its route. Yet, he continued, how interesting to see roads not seen before and get to know new people. The driver so polite and helpful.

Was it painful?

Being shut in the mask was 'hell', he said.

He'd used the word only once before. When, after the corner of a car door pierced his eye in Edinburgh, doctors bandaged it up to heal. (Mother and I took the car back to Queensferry, neither knowing how to drive. We lurched down the streets together, swinging between gears and pedals, provoking vivid abuse.) Following 11 days of grit and anxiety and (we learnt) agony, the bandages were removed, and all his septic eye fell out. 'I've been in hell,' Father told Mother and me then.

Later, having lost balance, he stepped to the right of a ferry crossing the Forth, and gashed the side of his face. Left with one scarred working eye. He used it to its glorious full for 50 uncomplaining years.

Almost at his century, he was still driving very carefully round East Anglia.

'I've never had an accident,' he always replied when I suggested he might stop.

Perhaps not – but his stately pace drove other motorists mad.

'If you *were* in an accident, even if it wasn't your fault,' I said, 'a man of 96 with one scarred eye and a wonky knee would be blamed, however careful he'd been.'

'Face that if it happens,' he said. 'No need to anticipate.'

But daughter C and I did anticipate, and one autumn day we drove the car away. He looked so sadly after it we almost turned back.

8 December, Thursday

Out of the house by 7.15, that 'uncertain hour before the morning/ Near the ending of interminable night'. The town, gently breathing as I watched it in the early hours, is stirring now.

In the hospital we're again confused. 'This way,' I say. 'No this,' D says.

We're both wrong. We know we're right when we spy the brightly coloured pictures, then the poem on riding a bicycle written all along the wall, like the mouse's tale in *Alice in Wonderland*. About remembered joy and energy and young breath in the hair and a boy and girl together on the bike, with a little dog barking at them from behind his gate. Happiness and youth.

Bit tactless at the entrance to radio-onc.

We sit in white electric glare. Milton's 'darkness visible', Eliot's 'light invisible'. Just cruel. Occasionally I catch another patient's eye. We turn away. All of us a little shabby. Keep things loose and cotton, they're burning you, treat it like a burn

The Laura Ashley skirt reaches my ankles. It's uneven because hitched up round my waist with the knicker elastic.

In the washroom mirror I see my hair suits the red skirt, a sort of unkempt bob like a mop wig. A line of grey vest on the top of my tight jumper completes the picture. My inner bag-lady is out.

I emerge and sit down to wait. Smug in my new honesty, I still rebuke myself for not trying: for not fussing myself up with a little lipstick, some dangling ear-rings and a coloured scarf. Why am I in these 'fucked-up clothes' as the uninhibited young would say?

A fat schoolgirl, I was sent money from Ceylon to buy a civilian outfit. Without trying them on, I chose a felt sky-blue circle skirt, a

bright yellow zipped top and red elasticated belt. At 18, fat fell off
– au pairing does that to young foreign girls in provincial France –
and in Paris I borrowed money for a neat, buttoned, grey coat from
Printemps. I thought I looked chic; I turned round and round in the
shop mirror. The French assistants sniggered. Unfair, for the coat
caught glances on the Pont Neuf, if only from American preppies
trying to seem bohemian for a few gorgeous French weeks.

The magazines in the side waiting-room tell of celebs or cars. I begin
reading the only book I can find on my new mobile phone. *White
Fang* by Jack London. It's about a wolf and a man who'll be eaten
in a wild, ethical way. There's silence except for occasional radio-
people passing. They avert eyes in case we try to catch them and ask
where we are in the queue. Time is moving along; we're all overdue.

   Into the silence steps my glamorous friend H, whom I met in a
book club so heterogeneous and chatty we rarely had time to speak
of books. Now researching in Hospital-land. Dressed in smart professional garb, short well-cut skirt, glossy black high heels, neatly combed
hair, subtle make-up. My status rises as she speaks to me. We do a
little public chat. I try to move to social mode. She passes on before
I quite achieve it. Afterwards, a pleasant couple smile and nod to me.
They're from Bury. They travel an hour each way.

   I return to *White Fang*.

Back to the patients' lavatory. A lock in the middle of the door rather
than the edge, the door itself swings in and out. Inconvenient when
you're in a hurry. The washbasin is low, for dwarves. The fierce
insistence on hygiene makes everything look dirty. I stare in the
mirror, the light being sharper than at home. I have a moment of
non-recognition, forgetting to smile in defence, as one should if not
raised a beauty. I come out, dizzily disorientated.

   Where was I sitting? Am I sitting there already? We're all starting to look the same. Is this a senior moment? Dementia? (Let that fear fade – no time for a slow, diminishing disease.)

Would I recognise myself if I were looking at her/me on that seat? So nondescript. Worth making a noise at letting so common-place a Me go puff and out? A puff of dust? Wordsworth first wrote, 'The mind of man is framed even like the breath./ And harmony of music.' Older, he rewrote this beginning: 'Dust as we are . . .'

I've always found dust warm, fleetingly assertive too.

This random quoting isn't 'being kind to the Self'. Over my hot, agitating summer, as pain and heaviness accelerated and as (I now know) cancer cells proliferated and while I tried and failed to enter Hospital-land, I turned to self-help books. Squatting by shelves in the local bookshop, where you can browse undisturbed in quiet booths. At first too thrifty to buy; later disinclined, discovering each volume said much the same.

'Love yourself unconditionally.'

'Being kind to yourself results in significant physical, mental and emotional health benefits.' 'Self-worth' seems the thing, not out-moded 'self-respect'.

Does every 'Self' deserve kindness? If so, how do you do it? Show me in diagram form.

If it doesn't come naturally, can you dress the Self in red high heels and fishnet tights, then abuse it – a delicious masochism to cheer it up?

I pass by the desk to get a new treatment print-out. In Lilliputian type. The Rosetta Stone not more opaque. Or is it my new varifocals from Vision Express failing to focus? I lift them off to try reading from an angle, closing one lazy eye.

My time for today is 7.48. Such crazy precision. We're already way off schedule. *White Fang* isn't engrossing. Bitterness wells up like phlegm. It's been so very long since it all began. I want to talk about it – about me and all my cancers, all the medical fumblings. I want people to listen, knowing full well they have no reason. Why ever should they? We all go wrong some time, nothing special there.

I'm called by my first name, a name I intensely dislike. How have I dwindled? Should I protest – or is it apt only when the offender's a man? Does my uneven red skirt cause the informality? (In truth, it's my own fault: some women gave their name as *Mrs* So-and-So. I like Ms but it never really caught on in England – means 'divorced' said the woman in the bank. Other titles are out of place in Hospital-land: one's a Body, not a mind. If you said *Dr*, they'd ask if you were a medical doctor? No? Well then.) Having been summoned, I prepare for entry to the machine.

I'm told merely to move from one set of seats to another. For comfort I take from my bag a forest postcard from friend S in America, but fail to concentrate. I want to escape but am past imagining a road through trees and over hills.

As time passes I slump a little more. Some pages of *White Fang* and in at last. But on LA1. What's the problem with LA8? That's *my* machine, my own killing – whoops, healing – machine.

The girls ask pleasantly how I am. Fine, I intend to say. 'I'm tired.'

Drink more, says one of them.

Drink more? Do they have cast-iron bladders? Poor bladder, poor bowels. What Joker created this perverse anatomy?

Why oh why oh why, as we used to drawl in school. Why oh why oh why? Not so much 'Why me?' as just 'Why?' (You don't have to say this with colds or cholera.)

Pummelled into pain in the tailbone, then under the beam, the square eye, I'm meat again. 'By the shores of Gitche Gumee. By the shining

Big-Sea Water.' My first cloth book. Why has it come back now, jingling and jangling through my mind? I never liked it. Never cared for Hiawatha or Nokomis or wampum.

A whole adult life reading good writing, by Joyce, Yeats and Eliots (George and T.S.), and *in extremis* what pops into my burning mind is this doggerel. Why am I lumbered with such gauche baggage? If I must suffer the entanglements of literature, why are the nearest threads these clunking ones? Why can't I grab Keats's dead hand as it stretches towards me, or feel the scratch of Jane Austen's final pencil as she composes daft verses propped up in a rented Winchester bed?

When alone, I notice the music's turned off. The silence is dark and 'dark is a way and light is a place'. Dylan T's poems were my form prize at Dotheboys Hall. The book had the school crest on the front; I had to walk up on the stage to take it from the small, thin, frightening headmistress in peacock shawl, a parrot among crows. She gave me an ambiguous smile as she handed it over.

But what luxuriance in that book, what endearing ostentation.

9 December, Friday

The appointment's later today. Way down in the afternoon. There's to be a review. I wake definitively at 5 and await the time when the irritatingly bass voice announces we're joining Radio 4, then on comes the Shipping Forecast. I try to anticipate each inshore water as we go round the islands, or the 'archipelago' as it's fashionable to call it. Ardnamurchan Point to Cape Wrath including the Outer Hebrides. 'Rain later, good, occasionally poor.' I like the early morning programmes as the World Service morphs into Radio 4. The raucous end of the evening's another matter. The dreadful 'National' Anthem.

The sounds of morning in the road and in the kitchen.

The hospital's bustling. Maybe because of this, D and I lose our way again, forgetting the artwork, the scenes of Cornwall and Cumberland, the scruffy spindly Quentin Blake cartoons, children as spacemen. At last we reach the bicycle poem. I notice our clinic is called Emmeline.

Feminism. How wonderfully blunt and old-fashioned our old sort now seems, like Emmeline's herself. Neuroscience demolishing what we spent so much effort making, to dent that thousand-year-old binary.

Don't destroy difference, make the most of it, release your feminine superpowers for greater impact. Difference everywhere all over again.

What will neuroscience not re-make? Sexism, ageism, racism, classism: I fear it do the isms in different voices.

Yet, half a century back, how heady was my first brush with feminism American-style. Once tear-gas settled on the Vietnam War and draft-dodging chaps lost their glamour – Stokely Carmichael's famous quip that women's place in radical movements was 'prone'. Excited colourful women sitting in Florida in balmy weather acquainting ourselves – not an ounce of self-mockery – with the vulva and its secret folds. The corn goddess, invoked in candlelit seances on green beanbags, turning out as useless for good luck (or good health in my case) as the BVM or the wonderfully titled 'Lady-Unique-Inclination-of-the-Night'.

Better the jujus I wore round my neck in northern Ghana. One pupil with the best juju was bullied. She said she'd show us all: she made rain in a once clear sky. Truly so. She asked me to wear her juju in her exam time; I didn't quibble.

What might I have done with my life if I'd held on to her juju?

I think of those bright-eyed children from the mud huts. Did any pass the external London 'O level' exams? The new Akosombo Dam flooded acres and roads and ancestors, and the mammy truck with the scripts never arrived down south.

So they said.

The British Council in Accra sent up a comic film about aristocratic birthright, *Kind Hearts and Coronets*, for me to show the Kusasi and Mamprusi children in the open air — children who'd run from classrooms with spears to fight the old tribal fight. Those children knew a thing or two about inheritance.

3 years ago, with Cancer 1, S and I lit 6 candles to the BVM at the bleak shrine of Walsingham in Norfolk. Again in Venice's San Marco for Cancer 2. Now in America, S lights candles once more. I fear we're not catching the Blessed Ear.

More people in the waiting areas. I'm not so special today. Time passes. We sit. It seems *my* machine has broken or is on strike. What is it with LA8? Misty disappointment hangs in the room.

Seeing my glum response, one girl says she'd wanted to put eyes on the front of LA8 to personalise it, but this had been 'frowned upon'.

At last I'm called to LA1. I climb on to the high bench and watch the square eye.

I can't repress Gitche Gumee. I should use this unreading time to imprint a language, conjugate irregular Italian verbs. But the future seems dim and Italian gestures too alien. So I lie here splashing in Big-Sea Water. Can't even properly access the meretricious lines I copied into my 5-year diary as wit and wisdom.

Jane Austen mocked the habit when she stocked her heroine Catherine's mind with 'those quotations which are so serviceable and so soothing in the vicissitudes of eventful lives'. If my teen-aged self hadn't given up on *Northanger Abbey*, I might have been laughed out of this comical memorising of bite-sized insights. Recently I discovered that nugget-reading, if not collecting, is a family inheritance. The grandfather I never knew left Father his little book, *Be of Good Cheer*, from 'The Quiet Hour Series'. 'Take what is; trust what may be: that's life's lesson', according to Robert Browning and, perhaps more usefully in my grandfather's sad circumstances, 'The burden which was thoughtlessly got must be patiently carried.' What other sayings did he carry to the long disease-ridden siege of Ladysmith, to the Khyber Pass and Northwest Frontier, to the gas-polluted trenches of Flanders?

I'm bombarded by protons. The skin tries its best but can't cope. Elasticity – Austen's great word for the admirable mind and body – is gone. The pelvis is quiet, taut, reddening with each new day. It's burning. I try creams, aloe vera, even Greek yoghurt. Only time is elastic.

Are the cancer cells cringing and cowering? Are the others? How much of me can go before I'm not?

The girls leave the room but my head stays here, unprotected. Why don't they take my head with them out of harm's way – or provide a helmet? What must these rays be doing to its modest endowments? All of me is being burnt.

I think of Father and his ordeals. Once again, I feel weak with shame and pity.

Drink more, they say when they return. Their mantra. If you drink more, you pee more, and that, dear ladies, is the problem.

And the fatigue. 'It shouldn't be there yet,' says one of them. (Why can't I remember their names? I must appear discourteous.) Drink more. Pee more.

Settle down in the lav with a bottle of pop.

*

I'm back on the chairs waiting for my review. I wait 2 and a half hours.

By now almost everyone has left.

Finally, I see the reviewer, a sympathetic lady, Ms M. I don't want facile sympathy, or want it too much. I moan about jovial Consultant X (whom I'd like to murder but best keep that to myself in here), the delays I'm sure have landed me in this predicament. A whole summer of silent incompetence. (What else to blame for moving from bladder to uterus to vagina – or wherever the cancer's been chewing like a witch's foetus? What word is right: growing, eating, devouring, invading, destroying, colonising, cohabiting?)

Cancer is a Crab, the devil insect in Gillray's picture of gout. Arrow tail and four-fingered hands, claws digging into the fleshy foot, making pain.

Ms M seems to agree. I don't like it. I want opposition. I want to be wrong. I want her to tell me not to say a single word against Consultant X who is always right and who cannot be judged by someone as medically ignorant as I am, as me – or 'myself' as people say nowadays.

Her pity makes me garrulous. She believes gentle yoga, positive thinking, meditation and Indian massages might help.

With what exactly? Do they cure cancer?

No. So?

12 December, Monday

There's a friendly breast patient in the early morning slot. With short growing-out chemo hair, 40s perhaps, thin, pretty. I feel competitive, sitting on a high horse in illness chic. (Just as well there're no Stage

4 people here to overtop me.) What's this urge to push myself forward so grotesquely?

I was top of the class when I dropped Physics in Dotheboys Hall, and the list was read out at the end of every term. It gave me half a second's pleasure. No salve for the ignominy of F set for games, the very bottom – just me and the surly Welsh-speaking day girls in the rain on the slanting hillside with dripping lacrosse sticks. The humiliation second only to having your weight yelled out across the gym at the start of each school year – 'duw anwyl, 10 stone!' It's always about the body. Descartes, who took the mind as king, was *so* wrong.

Don't talk to me of cancer 'Stages' and 'Grades'. I see my fat, asthmatic, short-sighted early self struggle through years to arrive here.

'This long disease, my life.' Little crooked Alexander Pope knew how it felt. And he with consolation or curse of being an infant 'dipt in ink' who 'lisp'd in numbers'. Pleasant to think of the glittering verses of this 'Wasp of Twickenham', finding now they diminish self-pity. 'To live and die is all I have to do,' he wrote – between the two be 'social, cheerful, and serene'. Good to know yourself the master of your craft, as he did. Envy shrinks before the *truly* wonderful. It's the just-a-bit-better that knocks you flat.

(How fortunate I never met Pope to be mocked as a 'maudlin Poetess' or 'hireling Scribbler'.)

'How long have you been coming here?' asks a fellow patient.

I have more than double your sessions.

Your first cancer?

This is my third.

'Do you go to the Macmillan clinic to share?'

I don't. I don't really want gritty good cheer. Just snakes and ladders. You get better, you get worse, no rhyme or reason.

'They give you coffee and biscuits at the clinic,' she adds.
'What sort of biscuits?'

I'm uneasy when hospitals and public places mimic 'home'. When Radio 4 pretends to be your 'Aunty'.

I go in first to LA8. Deft now with boots, skirt and knickers. A friend from Scotland writes that when she went through something like this she gave up underwear altogether, 'nae knickers', she says. To be frank, this is me at home under the tent skirt, but too risky here or at work.

Silence on the slab except for the peeping machine tune. Deep silence between sounds.
  'All shall be well, and all shall be well, and all manner of thing shall be well,' as God said to blessed Julian immured in her cold Norwich cell. She murmured it to T. S. Eliot, who garbled it. You can't pass on a revelation, said Tom Paine.
  What manner of thing am I to become well?

Back home and on to the Web. 80% should get better, 20% should not. 20%. But 40% have radiation sickness. And bowels packing up. I don't go further into it. No stages and grades, nothing specific. I push myself off, close down the computer.

I have to exaggerate to make a point, to make a possibility of things turning out just a little better than I fear.

I try to do something in the office. I've laid aside my red floppy skirt and put on a black long evening one that will do duty for the old sleek trousers. Am I sufficiently disguised? Hidden or not, I'm too fuzzy headed to be much use, tired of being tired. My colleagues are professionalising our workplace, weeding out dodos. The sick too? In this 'going-forward' world of work, they must look askance at me. Amiable colleagues, but still.

The healthy believe people are ill or well, the sick see a menacing cline. The well are smug, thinking they deserve vigour and good luck: the sick doubt, but should keep mum. Which are the more banal?

That I go into the office at all is a type of vanity. Oh, I know that.

I ring Father in his flat by the park. He talks about Christmas, what he should get for C's Baby who already has everything. He wonders what spring bulbs have been put in the empty flowerbeds. He hopes there'll be purple tulips.

I cut him short, pretending to hear a doorbell.

13 December, Tuesday

The morning is darker. And moister. I'm on my own. A low feeling in the waiting area despite Christmas tinsel. I think about teleology. When a clock goes tic tic we hear tic toc. There must be progress and where there's progress there must be an end. Where there's life, there must be death. But not the reverse. Can't get a tic out of a toc.

I should justify this writing with something halfway profound, but that's as far as old fuzzy brain can go. Terry Waite, the hostage kept for years in solitary confinement in Beirut, later blamed himself for having 'no great thoughts' during his imprisonment. All I can grasp is that everything is survivable except death.

I'm called in to the machine before I've read even a page of *White Fang* or exchanged pleasantries with the Bury couple. Looking at the square eye, cotton knickers drawn down to reveal increasing bareness.

Next year may include my death, I melodramatise. Why not? I'm an only child, a unique: such a one has no audience, no one to take her down a peg or 2, or buck her up. No one to practise projecting nice- ness with or try out appealing gestures before unleashing herself on a new world.

Young Jane Austen and Dickens and the Brontës amused siblings with their stories, exhibited themselves to please and entertain. It shows. An only child can only entertain herself. Using the comic mode, if ever, in most intense fashion. Only children don't do irony well: they do melodrama. Self-creation, not self-contrivance. They have difficulty telling which story they're in at any time. (I'm no academic in Hospital-land, so have licence to generalise.)

Christmas music in the room. I can't sing along – no one sings on a bier. In any case, at best of times, I sing poorly. Here comes Dotheboys Hall again. Oh this dredging, meandering pelvic memory. Digging up 'old, unhappy far-off things'.

Why is this school brushing against me like this? Poking and prodding when I thought I'd done with it.

Because the first 20 years swallow memories and other years regur- gitate? I fear so – from reading or living.

Because I'm deprived of words? Like then. That too.

In my first year, sour matron confiscated my under-the-blanket black- and-red torch and left me with my own mind for company.

Never much fun, especially when you're 11 and in exile.

Odd way with words in that school. Does anyone outside Wales do choral speaking? 'Come back!' cried the lighthouse keeper, for God's sake girls come back!' Or 'Hid by the surge's swell, / The

Mariners heard the warning bell; / And then they knew the perilous rock, / And blessed the Abbot of Aberbrothok.' Something of the sort. 'The Dong with the Luminous Nose', the 's' being a hiss in our halted accent.

There's wisdom for you: girls keeping warm by dramatic speaking and friction from green prickly best-dresses.

My mind's furring up along its connectives. This is a side-effect, says the Macmillan pamphlet. And my bladder?

Lacks stamina.

A Scottish friend sends a recipe she says works for a low-residue diet and helps the immune system. I look it over: all crimson. 2 red onions quartered, 2 tomatoes, 2 red peppers, seeded and quartered, 2 carrots, in large chunks, 2 beetroot, quartered, 2 – 4 cloves of garlic, lightly smashed, 1 to 1.5 litres vegetable stock. Garnish with chopped pumpkin seeds.

Lentils and tomatoes and pumpkin seeds?? On what robust planet is she living? The immune system indeed. I have more important things to worry about than immunity.

14 December, Wednesday

Celebrated invalids with private means revel in admitting visitors and voyeurs to their bedside, holding court in flower-scented boudoirs. Not being celebrated, I want no visitors. But it moves me that D's in the kitchen in the early morning dark making a Victoria sponge for me, the lovely smell mounting the stairs to form a warm blanket in the attic bedroom. Such a generous thing. How dare Jane A mock 'the purchase of a sponge-cake'! Who said the smell of a pancake is a better motive for staying in this world than any senti-mental reason?

We leave the cake cooling on a rack, then off in the dark. The same car-park space as yesterday.

Trail along the corridors, gloom lolloping along beside.

When we arrive, prostates are drinking ice-cold water. I don't have to. I know that now. This is a pre-feminist, gendered space: here the body's no cultural construction. Women pelvics don't have to drink ice water. (Indeed better not.)

Do the girls look at us and think: we will be like them – or doubt they ever can be?

'As we are now so will you be,' written over the Norfolk alms-houses where the decrepit lived to be gawped at by the young and hale. The terrible progress from cuteness to this.

Anti-ageing products cluttering shops. Anti-dying creams?

Nothing like old age and disease to teach you that you really *aren't* worth it.

Only a little wait and on to LA8. Will it become a friend? It concentrates only on me, like the therapist with her minimal needs I like to imagine dissolving all hurts, or an over-fond mother confessor sucking off feebleness and guilt. (Regretting the waste of those years in North America with an insurance policy that paid for psycho-analysis but not for dentistry – and I with my rotten ration-book teeth.) The tailbone is jammed on to the slab, legs in uncouth angle.

Count it down. Count. Numbers always solace and release (unless they form percentages). Count the sheep, the stairs, the letters, the breaths. Just keep counting. Count out Dotheboys Hall, that place I had no business to be in.

But no, it's not to be done.

I numbered the days and months and years till Mother and Father would sail in to take me away. I turned the years into minutes, minutes into seconds. Good for maths but not for insomnia. For that I had to stop the snoring and snuffling from the next beds. I persuaded the girls to tell plots of films they saw in the holidays. But they fell asleep before finishing. Only I left conscious. I tried to wake them and they didn't like it.

Plump and (just then) tall for my age, I was the first in that dormitory to have a period. An unexpected event when things like this weren't talked about by mother and daughter. Matron threw a packet of sanitary towels on to the bed. By the evening they were hanging like a ribbon of sausages from the light flex.

Before getting into bed, we each knelt on the cold linoleum floor to say prayers. We were to pray for family, then friends, then for ourselves, that we would avoid sins the next day. I prayed with fervour: 'Get me out of here, oh Lord, now. Use any means.'

I spent the rest of the cold night hours planning the journey overland from Wales through mountains and deserts and down major rivers to Ceylon, changing clothes as I changed zones. I knew all the cities between Calais and Pondicherry and the kind of transport – train, ferry, bus, boat, camel, rickshaw, catamaran – most likely to take me onwards. Such knowledge of little use when told for 'O level' Geography to mark on the map the coal mines of South Wales, and describe the physical terrain round Princes Risborough.

The imagined journey stuck in my mind like a diamond in a ring. As if I'd taken it on Aladdin's magic carpet.

*

WJEC was the hardest exam board – they said: Wales always tried hardest, having the most to prove. Victorian Blue Books declared Welsh children more stupid than their English counterparts. The Welsh language was evasive: it had been the language of slavery.

They meant to do right by me, my clever, uneducated parents. With no failure of heart but with no notion how an 11-year-old would be jolted to find herself 6,000 miles from home. (Father would have coped, perhaps not Mother.) Loving enough, as parents were in those days, but emotionally squeamish about discussing or anticipating what might be felt. Self-censorship still a virtue in the 1950s.

Their choice had to fall on Wales: I might be kept in school for half-terms, but must be parked somewhere in holidays. Only Aunty available. So, no chance of those gracious costly schools like Cheltenham Ladies or Roedean or Dartington that educated and 'finished' a girl with sophistication, self-possession, and manners as well as learning – so I thought later.

They couldn't know about elite schools. But they *should* have noticed that North Wales was Welsh-speaking where our middle part was not.

They found the place in a catalogue which provided one black-and-white photo for each boarding school. The Welsh one was out of focus, bleak, looking like the Classic Comics version of Wuthering Heights. Its motto *Ardua Semper* gave away nothing: neither of them knew Latin.

In the event I needed only Welsh basics: *cachau bant, cau dy geg, mochyn budr* – I think. A form of protest not to learn more – and no lessons on offer for us monolinguals. Now, knowing a little of those glittering, flaming poets like Taliesin and Aneirin and naughty, ogling Dafydd ap Gwilym, I wish I'd had the chance (and desire) to learn.

*

My Welsh phrases cut no mustard in my next, posher school near London – and my Welsh accent had the girls rolling eyes. Unusually, Mother had failed to insert me into the local state school. The drunk teacher in Ceylon had, it emerged, lost my answers to the Moray House Test taken many years before in lieu of the 11-Plus (we'd been told); no state 6th form would have me.

I wasn't in the posh one long enough to run up much expense. Soon I was selling gentlemen's underwear in Marks & Sparks. There when I heard I'd got a place at Cambridge.

Some comfort, since Mother and I had just emerged from a confidence trick.

An elderly lady, supposedly a professor at London University – she had the stripy scarf and some crested books – struck up an acquaintance with Father; then, through him, presented me with a Latin dictionary (maybe he mentioned I hated the subject with its rigmarole of tortoises and phalanxes?). The woman was called Nella Hooker – how could we be so innocent?

She told Mother I must go to Oxford and the only way was through influence – hers. We believed her! (Mother was initially dubious, but she'd read that the ratio of boys to girls at Oxford was much in favour of girls getting married to a doctor or lawyer from 'nice' people – as well as being educated – so she came round to the idea. Marriage was an urgency in 1960.)

In pursuit of the unexpected goal, she entertained Mrs H with fish and meat pies over many months while I was persuaded, much against inclination, to visit her for tea on Sundays. She gave us fine gifts of beaded bags and Victorian fans – looking like items from a museum, as they undoubtedly were. One day she dragged me to Oxford, pointed out a college and said she knew the principal. Looking back, I think it was St Hugh's but could just as well have been a school or borstal.

Then we went into expensive shops where she 'bought' me books and trinkets – always saying she'd paid for them as I left clutching the unwrapped things.

Finally we learnt just a bit of the truth through dedicated sleuthing – Mother kept meticulous notes – among grand, rich people (her relatives?), who rather ominously warned us to be very afraid before they slammed their doors and told us never to return. She'd spent time in Holloway Prison but the police were cagey about giving out information. When we confronted her, we received abuse and a parting shot that I would never ever have got into Oxford, not even with the Queen and Archbishop of Canterbury as referees.

What was it for? We never knew. We had no money, nothing to tempt a professional confidence trickster to take such trouble, to make such elaborate pretences – we met people supposed to be titled while we in turn were passed off as Lady X and her daughter! Mother suggested 'white slavery', since Mrs H seemed to have another teen-aged girl in tow, but, with a rather Turkish-harem notion of this, I thought it too glamorous. She was probably trying to get me caught for shop-lifting: this would have put me in her power perhaps, but to what end?

Now I'm old, I wonder if she simply saw comfort in our home and, after a hustling life, wanted a berth. But what was all that about Oxford?

Working in a new unfamiliar job, Father was largely absent from the finale of the saga. When Mother and I laid out to him incontrovertible proof, he was at first incredulous, then remarked, 'The poor woman must have been very unhappy.' Since one of Mrs H's parting shots was that Father was too good for both of us, Mother sniffed at this. He hadn't had to do the cooking or endure Sunday teas.

All this Oxford talk had fired me up for Cambridge; so, I became an external candidate.

I had no school to tell me how things were done. At the point when I should have heard the result of the exam and interview, Mother received a telegram. She phoned M&S. The ring sounded way over the counters. The supervisor was saying, 'The girls aren't allowed private calls,' as I dashed into her. 'Please,' I said, 'it might be.' She gave in – I was no great sales assistant, perhaps she felt sorry for me.

'It's a telegram,' said Mother. 'It says "Vacancy Newnham". What do you think it means?'

'I don't know,' I said rather crushed. 'But would they have sent a telegram if they didn't mean I was in?'

'Funny way of saying it,' said Mother.

I was suddenly sure. Head over heels in love with the idea of Cambridge because John Milton had been there – even though girls weren't allowed into *his* college.

Jolly lucky to be accepted since my method of preparing for the entrance exam had been to memorise my magpie hoard of quotations about Life in the 5-year diary. Fortunately, the questions gave little scope for disgorging them.

From my perspective, interviews were equally eccentric: at Girton College I was asked about the Beat Poets of whom I'd never heard. Not a word about Milton. I found that perplexing.

'I've no idea what's going on,' I remember saying to the final interviewer from Newnham. (Not unlike the previous year with Nella Hooker.)

'Never mind,' said Mother when I got home, having missed the train connection at Bletchley. 'Your interview suit will always be useful.'

With his cheery temperament, Father had been sanguine, though ready for Plan B if Plan A failed. He cared nothing about marriage prospects at Cambridge but, when Mother told him the news, became wildly excited. He came home early, bearing the *Shorter Oxford English*

Dictionary in 2 volumes, as well as a jar of candied ginger tied in red ribbon and a piece of wonderful German cheesecake: it had just become a delicacy in English shops.

Mother remarked that the English dictionaries replaced the unwelcome Latin one that began the Nella episode. (She was defensive because she'd managed to lose the telegram.)

In my Cambridge years I didn't visit Milton's college, having understood he was no longer fashionable among the critically sophisticated (despite writing the best last lines ever in *Paradise Lost*), that the *life* of an author was irrelevant, and that the Cam was not now as 'sedgy' as when he'd so thrillingly described it.

I had no occasion to wear my interview suit again: no student would be seen dead in such a costume after 1960.

My time in M&S was well spent. I learnt that girls on lingerie and sportswear were cleverer than me with my education in regurgitating – from Latin to Biology – and that our insulting educational system needed overhauling. If I'd read carefully, I'd have got this from Jane Austen, with her robust contempt for traditional schooling, but warm regard for moral, social training. Sadly, it was years before she and I became intimate. ('Clever' was, I gathered at Cambridge, a slightly denigrating term for the quick and shallow – the coveted word was 'brilliant' – usually applied to boys of 18 from public schools or left-wing, argumentative homes. I was never 'brilliant'. In America looking for jobs, I sold my Cambridge years with F.R. and Q.D. Leavis, Raymond Williams and visiting C.S. Lewis, when in truth I learnt more in smoke-filled seminars in Florida, being ready at last to listen and be prodded over the cliff. Besides, by then I'd read the book that changed everything, Kate Millett's *Sexual Politics,* which told me I need not find only greatness in language that also screamed misogyny.)

*

The idiots are cocksure, the intelligent are full of doubt, said Bertrand Russell, getting it not quite right. (How could he with that posh background and white, godlike hair?) Better the French essayist, Montaigne, who never made it into my teen-age book of snippets: 'It is a disaster that wisdom forbids you to be satisfied with yourself and always sends you away dissatisfied and fearful, whereas stubbornness and foolhardiness fill their hosts with joy and assurance.' Long-winded but true.

Bertrand Russell also said, when in his 90s, that, if he could live his life again, he would. The same life or another one? If the first, he must be mad or insensitive. Did he forget the pain of Sisyphus, pushing that rock over and over, knowing the end?

They are not long the days of wine and roses: not everyone quaffs and sniffs with intensity. But a few extra years now, even so diminished, yes please – or I wouldn't be here, so avid for what I might miss. I don't mean joining 'the choir invisible' either. I mean just being here in the most ordinary way. Yes, please.

I have some good memories – see, getting that telegram from Newnham – then, later, gazing round its pretty library; the sleuthing with Mother was fun, so was drinking palm wine in mud compounds in northern Ghana, grabbing at flying fish in Ceylon, carrying Aunty's pink blancmange rabbit and green splattered jelly to the Baptist social, mushrooming with old Father in the woods among drying leaves, watching our black dog leaping over the long grass across the road in Bermuda, skinny-dipping in the Pine Barrens, returning to a clapboard house through a sunset of wild pollution. (Memories always tend to the superlative.)

Books too gratify in memory. And, unlike my own constructed ones, *their* images never make me squirm. They come wrapped in gorgeous style – even the gargantuan feast of Dmitri and Grushenka or the fiery visceral pains of Satan. (If Milton had been my poetic teen-aged passion, the *novelist* of choice was always Dostoevsky. Neither much use in the quotidian, it must be said.)

I'd like to root around and make some more memories in life and books before the final trip to Hospital-land. Not be stuck in this museum.

Today, despite silently counting and chanting, remembering some things, trying to forget others, I feel my buttocks most painfully splayed; the machine especially violent.

Date of birth? I'm asked every morning. My identity. No chance of slicing off a few years, as women used to do, the Empress Josephine and Emma Hamilton for starters.

'At your age,' they said to Father just the other day in this hospital. At your age: they mean, 'Is it worth it?'

In Puerto Rico where C was born among pregnant women screaming for the Virgin, identity was a footprint on the birth certificate.

My friends in America say I'm having radiation because chemo is more expensive. Americans know medical terms and use them without embarrassment. They keep a check on the body and its treatments. They know their blood group and pressure and their cholesterol. I don't even know what 'metastasis' means or what a 'stent' is. Or a 'fistula'. A French friend says, you want brachytherapy but I expect that's too much for your NHS. I hope, says another American, you've had a second opinion, and a third if needs be.

Ah yes, that Second Opinion, that Choice of hospitals and procedures the government promised? Where exactly? Don't thieves and doctors stick together? (I know: aggression's a form of panic.) In any case by the time we'd motored round the country trying to find oncologists with free time, the crab would have grown its swollen legs clean out of my mouth.

Besides, there should be no criticism: the NHS is England, our patriotism.

*

Actually, when first hearing the term, I'd no more idea of the 'endo-metrium' than of a 'fistula'. (Was it real? In *The Doctor's Dilemma*, George Bernard Shaw lets his avaricious surgeon invent a nut-shaped abdominal organ called the 'nuciform sac'. It always demanded removal – if the patient had money. Like adenoids and tonsils when I was young, whipped out of childish throats before they could mutter Jack Robinson.) Turns out the endometrium is the lining of the womb. So, out it all came. No loss there. In the past an ageing womb had purpose, wandering round the body, bumping into organs, causing creative hysteria. Nothing so marvellous now.

Cancer cells are eternal. They cannibalise everything: munch, munch. Hair and nails were supposed to grow after death. Opening Lizzie Siddal's grave to get out the poems he buried with her in a grand but regretted gesture, Dante Gabriel Rossetti found her awash with red hair. So it was said, but it was a lie, an illusion caused by a shrunken skull. Cancer cells could burst the tomb and straggle over the yard like an unruly pumpkin vine.

I get back home so tired it's hard to mount the stairs. Into the lava-tory, side-effects definitely kicking in.

As I sit, I cheer myself by imagining the late breakfast. It will be good and surely stay in place for an hour or 2. White bread and pale butter just as the Macmillan booklet advises, jelly jam, no pips, no fibre residue.

Such white diet, approaching the realm of light. No sex, no body, no cancer. Just the female angel come to burn in the machine. Such purity in burning. Tears press my eyes when I think of all this purity. And myself chewing it quietly downstairs.

I'm still in the cubicle when the phone rings. I come out to answer. It's Father, poor old Father. Dreadful, he says, such pain, such misery.

He used to be so stoic but, at 99, at last it's too much. In agony since 4 in the morning. 'You should have rung 999,' I say. 'I rang you,' he says. I feel such sadness that he waited, and that I so want that white breakfast and won't have it.

D and I call a doctor but it's hours before Father's actually in hospital in a real bed, the formalities so strenuous and, despite blood and pain and age, he must wait his turn behind children with hurt fingers and unkempt men getting out of the cold.

The bowels are collapsing, he's in bad shape. I'm tired, so tired. D stays in hospital with him; I go home to get under the duvet, then into the lavatory.

I'm so used to poor Father cheering others along and telling stories of 'strange wonders that befell' him: I can't really believe I left him there in silence.

A few hours later. D and I are back in hospital. I take in a couple of public facilities on the way to Father's ward. Out of habit we almost go to the bicycle poem by Emmeline, but stop ourselves in time. He isn't where initially put. We find him in an overspill from Urology.

Lying in bed, he looks like a dead man with his one plastic eye awry, his mouth open – but he's breathing harshly. My friend H comes by, she looks grave. She expects him to die soon.

Why? Just because he's 99. It's no age, he says so often. Old Parr was 152 and he came from near Father's place, good healthy country air in the lungs. He loves Old Parr and tells the story of how he was dragged to London to see King Charles, was fed the rich wine and food he'd always eschewed, then promptly died.

Father enjoys red wine and good steak, so no change of fare, no reason to give up now.

*

I've seen him often on the brink and not tumbling over. One Boxing Day a few years back, already in his 90s, he was knocked clean down by a speeding car in King's Lynn. We were summoned to hospital, to the deathbed. He woke up and went home that day.

He's not so easily silenced. No more stories? All that energy and indignation and generosity and curiosity snuffed out? Unimaginable.

Sing in me, Muse, and through me proclaim the story of that man, the wanderer, harried for years, that man who, though buffeted, would never gaze out indifferently on the world.

When he wakes, he tells in some detail symptoms rather worse than my own but of the same genre.

Now we're both obsessed with shit, a transgressive word Father would never use, certainly not with a lady present. (What's the alternative? Toddler 'poo', pompous 'excrement' or comic 'ordure'?) Great conversation. Both think the other should be less forthcoming. We're disgusted with our interest, interested in our disgust. We recoil only from the other's products, no guts for other people's guts.

The selfishness of sickness is overwhelming. We've discarded other subjects – except the Baby, so long awaited. That alone perks up the failing, flailing mind. Yes, I say, absolutely. The best thing of all.

Back home there's now nothing I want to eat, not even the white breakfast or the Victoria sponge which goes stale before your eyes. Later I heat up a tinned sticky toffee pudding in the microwave. No fibre in that concatenation of sugar and fat. I eat one chemical spoonful and jettison the rest.

Father can't be dying. He hasn't in near 100 years.

15 December, Thursday

While exposing my flesh on the slab I mention the problems, and more. No need for detail. Take Imodium, the girls say (I wish I could remember their names – or read their tiny labels). I fear the advice: drugs can make things worse.

I stay in corpse pose as the machine only slowly begins to circum-navigate my dismal continent.

In Princeton with students amused that I, their teacher, despite years of communal living and tear-gas and protests with a husband looking like Che Guevara, had never sampled pot. I used not to admit this, like being a virgin in third year at college, which thanks to my au pairing I wasn't. So, I puffed. (Asthma ensured I was never a smoker.) Nothing happened, I puffed again and again. Then I reeled, panicked, and fell over. They panicked.

Poor students: a cry for help could eject them from their pleasant lodgings, but a dead professor would be more embarrassing. They summoned an ambulance. In the infirmary and fully awake, I was preparing a story when a young doctor told me not to bother. I'd over breathed and become anxious.

Yes, the students were evicted.

Then a stronger, more sophisticated drug. I'd come to England and met a man who was a great smoker of cigarettes and marijuana, imbiber of all transforming substances, a Marxist lover of Musil and Adorno. I admired the intellectual stance as much as I had, years before, the Che Guevara look – always a sucker for fierce Marxist men, however troubled their temperament. He gave a party, everyone smoked. I told the Princeton pot story. Eat it then, they said, and I did. I waited. And ate another bit. Looking like little chunks of plasticine.

Then the world tipped over. Pictures on the wall moved out and up-ended; trees and vines sprouted from frames and spilt like liquid across the floor. They put away the glasses and refroze the quiches: the party was over. The supplier from the yachts was cross, seeing no reason to end the fun. No doctor this time. Another little brush with death I thought, like the polio in Ceylon, the malaria and poisoned leg in Ghana.

The upside-down world lasted a full 24 hours. Swallowed by pink and red guilt. And I a mother.

Life so brief and fragile, best not tamper with it.

(If you want intoxication, try asthmatic insomnia nights, their entoptic and endaural flora.)

D and I leave radio-onc and go down towards the car park. A group of young employees trip past giggling. I marvel at their healthy insouciance and frown. Then the corridor slants in carnivalesque mode, like the pictures in the party house. I have a nosebleed. What other unruly effluents can there be? The modest symptoms of cancer pale beside the effects of malignant, medical 'cure'.

16 December, Friday

Only a 30-minute wait today. A couple of chapters of *White Fang* and his doggy adventures. A young girl coughs, sneezes and spits into a whole box of tissues. I edge away. I can't go on the machine if I catch cold. What happens if you sneeze into the eye? It would all be ruined. Mrs Bennet in *Pride and Prejudice* remarked, 'People do not die of little trifling colds.' But her daughter nearly did.

The radio girls are different. I'm told and promptly forget their names, distracted by the bright scarlet and pink hair of the shorter one. My professionalising colleagues repeat names on meeting, then use them often: that way they imprint memory, make friends and influence the world. I admire but can't emulate. Too old to learn tricks.

Fuzzing brain is chanting as I walk from the waiting seat to the machine's couch, 'God's in His heaven – All's right with the world!' Pippa's refrain in Browning's *Pippa Passes*.

Am I mumbling aloud?

I sometimes speak to ducks on the Cam's sluggish riverbank: I don't mimic or talk down to them.

Climbing on to my slab, I plan to control my mind. Prisoners in solitary confinement keep sane with useful memories. I poke and make random sparks. Either tinnitus or a fly is in the room. 'I heard a Fly buzz – when I died.'

'Rage against the dying of the light,' wordy Dylan said to his pa. Might work for a large man but not the best idea for a short woman. Like me and Mother.

An American colleague once remarked I was 'big on control'. Too right. Wouldn't need to be if I were a strapping 6-footer. I'd stride towards the sunset, silently outraged.

Personal size and emotions aren't congruent. Obese Mrs Musgrove in *Persuasion* shed real tears for her worthless dead son. An unbecoming conjunction which curled the handsome lips of hero and heroine. Good taste couldn't accommodate the sight. That's all I can do with sour Jane A – have you seen her face, her real face, not the one they put on souvenir tea-towels? Saint Jane indeed!

I love her books but not herself – so censorious, so acid, making us all into Mrs Eltons before the snobbish poise of Emma – who's in reality as 'vulgar' as her foe. (Imagine Pope and Austen at tea with you, imagine the mordant irony and crafty wit. Best be out of earshot once you inelegantly leave the room.)

In any case, Jane A can't keep raging Dylan – or Gitche Gumee – at bay.

As I morosely moved along corridors in New Jersey, yet another colleague in my department, with a large proportion of Jewish people, commented, 'You'd be better if you accepted your Jewishness.'

'But I'm not Jewish.'

He gave a knowing smile.

Why didn't I leap at the chance? Such a fine, warm, colourful, energetic identity to have in New York. I could have snuggled in with all those glorious women I worked with or briefly met, Adrienne Rich, Gloria Steinem, Marge Piercy, Marilyn French, Kate Stimpson and Elaine Showalter. In my many years in America, I never met a soul from mid-Wales.

Some whacky people think the Welsh are part of the 10 lost tribes of Israel. Whatever the case, for the American job market, I presented myself as *English*. I regard my accent as sub-RP, except when over-excited. My wonderful (Jewish) friend from Newnham, Miriam Margolyes, so attuned to voice, noticed the lilt in the higher register.

Why was I morose in that corridor? I liked teaching in the States very much, but never learnt its codes, having only scattered shards of understanding even after so many years (close friends were other 'resident aliens'). There seemed so little room for my sort of bristly irony and vigorous grumbling.

For a women's writing series, I compiled a book of interviews with English and American authors. On publication, I received a furious letter from May Sarton, who complained I'd made her less positive than she was. I thought I'd been admiring and sympathetic. I misjudged.

Better luck with Joan Barton from Salisbury, poet of concrete, precise verse. Philip Larkin and Walter de la Mare praised her early work. A land-girl and worker for the British Council during the war, laid off when men came home. In time she became a skilled dealer in second-hand books and returned to poetry. I liked her 'Thursday's Child' condemned to go far – I too was a Thursday's child – but mostly her poems are about meagre lives written into beauty. The one I included in the book came from her experience as a dealer: 'Lot 304: Various Books':

> There are always lives
> Left between the leaves
> Scattering as I dust
> The honeymoon edelweiss
> Pressed ferns from prayer-books
> Seed lists and hints on puddings
> Deprecatory letters from old cousins
> Proposing to come for Easter
> And always clouded negatives
> The ghost dogs in the vanishing gardens:
>
> Fading ephemera of non-events,
> Whoever owned it
> (Dead or cut adrift or homeless in a home)
> Nothing to me, a number, or if a name
> Then meaningless,
> Yet always as I touch a current flows,
> The poles connect, the wards latch into place,
> A life extends me—
> Love-hate; grief; faith; wonder;
> Tenderness.

In Salamanca old library, D and I visited an exhibition of things left inside books. One was a condom.

Joan Barton wasn't always positive in the way Americans are (to their benefit). Together we spoke of our escape in poetry and stories, their tentacles in the mind. Then we grumbled about the weather and ate scones.

Yet, despite this alienation, this moaning about American positivity – when I returned to England, I found myself a misfit. The accent I thought of and sold as English was in England heard as Transatlantic, while my lack of dignified reserve – speaking to strangers in library tearooms or probing, instead of ignoring, moods – was alien. As was my writing, my interest in women authors still unfashionable in English academia, my love of speculation as well as scholarship.

There should be a mid-Atlantic island for us mixed-culture oddities: somewhere near Bermuda. There, like those old 1790s radicals left living into a primmer 19th century – Hazlitt, Godwin, Holcroft and Thelwall, we could make 'seditious allegories' mocking all our cultures, our ill luck to be rootless.

Death too, now I come to think of it. All grist to an allegorical mill, the chance to say if cornered by culture or approaching death, 'What me? I meant no such offence.'

Death shall have no dominion, said Dylan T provocatively, knowing full well that it has.

The slightest movement on the hard bed will make the machine irradiate liver or fluttery heart – or mind, finishing off memory altogether, real and literary. Not an uplifting line, not a troublesome phrase left of wampum and spiring-spearing herons.

Of them all, Dylan Thomas sticks most (after Hiawatha), coming in when I was so young and being a comfort under the blanket. 'We are not wholly bad or good/Who live our lives under Milk Wood.' Better to share your bier with Dylan than Percy Bysshe. 'Death is the veil which those who live call life.' A young man's fantasy. 'We might be all We dream of happy, high, majestical.' Yes, yes, sigh. 'We are not wholly bad or good.'

Mother loved *Under Milk Wood*, Gossamer Beynon and Captain Cat, Willy Nilly Postman, little Polly Garter and Nogood Boyo rocking out in the bay.

I stare up, blinking with rambling tiredness. Am I on LA1 or LA8? I'm breathing normally. I wonder at the novelty. Neither holding my breath nor gulping.

For an asthmatic, to be ill and breathing is curious. Nothing so central as asthma. Nothing else loses you in breath. Nothing else takes your breath away without knocking you stone dead. (In my pious teen-age years, I accepted miseries as penalties, but asthma was enigmatic, an identity; I thought it my cross but never quite my punishment.)

So many diseases: dysentery more than once, polio suspected, malaria often, very bad measles, mumps and chicken pox and flus and colds and bronchitis more times than I can say, and blood and stomach bugs galore, infected sores that bloated my leg like a dead dog and took me into the world's worst hospital in Ghana where the latrines outdid the Great Stink of 1858 – but no, no going there – and chronic fatigue, osteoporosis, and coughs and catarrh of course, never free there. But nothing comes close to asthma at full throttle.

It arrived with me in a Welsh world of feather beds and coal fires in a damp, blacked-out attic with bulging wallpaper holding in dribbling plaster. Drink red wine, whisky, and off you go, smoke a cigarette, run too fast, have sex – yes, even that – feel a sudden chill wind, smell scent, polish, an air freshener, a dog on a chair, a rolled-up cat, a budgie in his cage, and the breath is caught and coarsened. Keats and his quiet breathing indeed; simple enough then to be half in love with 'easeful death'.

Asthmatics don't imagine easeful death. Keats was preposterous even for consumption; composing the words before he knew of real death. If Dylan T's pa seemed to rage, it would have been raucous breathing.

No nights like Welsh moorland nights before little Bakelite wirelesses and televisions and phones and lovely gadgets, and only the terrible wind breaking the silence by whining and hooting, banging its great undulating lungs against the ill-fitting window, then the white fingers entering the attic rooms through cracks round the frames, reaching whitely down into your mouth, making the breath hitch and rasp. You cannot shut your mouth for trying to breathe, for screaming. I think I gave up sleep then, at 2 or 3. Not worth the bother.

Cancer is no consumption, though clever Susan Sontag linked them as victims of our chronic urge to metaphor. Did anyone outside Stendhal's novels really avoid the word 'consumption' as they did 'cancer' when I was young? Spelling it out in whispered capitals: 'She has C A N C E R.' (Maybe they did: Kafka said people grew glassy-eyed when they had to mention TB.)

The differences are huge of course. Consumptives were thin – they call me Mimi – with ribs stuck together like grissini in a tight packet, making their transparent dying selves known by a single red spot on the whitest handkerchief. They could be chic, like La Dame aux Camélias. Consumption was passionate, hectic, loud, expressive (like asthma – though that disease never achieved poetry). Spiritual too, refined, sensitive. ('I should like to die of consumption,' said fat Byron.) Cancer's obscene, obese, repressive, a punishment of those who kept in anger and desire and whatever else should be let out – metaphorically, that is.

My mind returns to what is, alas, too much let out.

*

Putting things into words is putting them into the realm of reason, said Freud. I want to live there, quietly breathing in the realm of reason, thin but not too thin.

Cancer, I say firmly – proudly? Times have changed since Susan Sontag berated us for our secrecy and fear. Since W. H. Auden described repressed, thin-lipped and yearning Miss Gee growing cancer like an assassin inside her, but not telling till it was too late.

Asthma, I say, I have and always have had asthma. Doesn't have the same ring.

Words are relational. I know. But they existed for me and spoke to me by myself, no matter I was often ignorant of what they meant. Spending so much time alone – especially in those holidays when, except for deaf Aunty after work, I spoke to no one for days on end, tramping moorlands and hills in sub-Miltonic wordy daze (Wordsworth would have better served but, if Milton's in your head, you see thyme, willows and hazel copses).

Now, in company, I talk too much and interrupt: compensating for so many silent years.

I met Wordsworth later: he helped my turn from epic to lyric. I'd imagined retelling the great Miltonic tale in rollicking iambics, the journey of Adam and Eve wandering 'through *Eden*' on 'their solitary way'. But *they* weren't solitary – 2 of them – *my* epic would show a wanderer alone. Then I discovered Wordsworth had been there already: I took heart from his 'self-sufficing power of Solitude'. Under his influence I submitted verses to a magazine describing visionary hill walks on the Long Mynd.

Excruciating when I saw them in print. I tried to dampen Father's usual enthusiasm, but Mother understood and put away the copies.

2 or 3 times in the hospital facilities between radio-onc and the Treatment Centre on my way to see Father. He's ill and in pain for

sure, but not dying. He can't be. When D says we'll have a goose for Christmas, he starts on a story about his widowed mother making rook pie for her family, plucking each individual bird for its teeny bit of meat. How many rooks and how long did it take? He may be the only person alive to know and be able to calculate. He's the only person to make me feel young.

There was a goose club in the village, people paid in all year for Christmas, he says. Then his mother roasted it on a spit, the grease dripping into a huge glistening pan.

The rest of the year meat came from the pig they'd raised, killed, and salted to bacon and ham. Poor as they were, someone in the village was always poorer: part of their store must be taken round to the invalid or old.

Back home I hear on the news that Christopher Hitchens has 'lost his fight' with cancer at 62. With what weapons did he battle? In what war was he fighting? What tactics? Trench warfare? And against what? (I like a good metaphor, a cliché for that matter. But really, this bellicosity among canceristas is too much when the 'enemy' is yourself. Yet, I suppose there's some reason for this militaristic rhetoric: cancer is attacked by poison and nuclear machines, is always about to be conquered.)

Friends said C. Hitchens knew 3 words for our one, could articulate what was vague in others, was clever, vain and knowledgeable. So charming but also infuriating, screaming, hectoring, badgering. Not a mode open to women, however battling. Women must be emollient, soothe and please, even without aptitude. (A confusion that ended for me in a manic desire to please, with equal desire to annoy.)

I contemplate Christopher Hitchens. To smoke and drink, be so acclaimed, then snuff yourself out. All your own doing. He 'loses his battle', says the headline. Won, rather. He chose. I didn't, I haven't. It snuck up on me; he dared it to come.

*

I feel the warm tentacles of self-pity. Let me make a bonfire of my hurts and flame out. Or just eat another piece of stale Victoria sponge.

19 December, Monday

Under the machine, thinking of Aldous Huxley in *Eyeless in Gaza* – Milton was blind when he wrote the phrase in *Samson Agonistes*. Aldous lifted it perhaps because he too was nearly blind – too much mescaline? His characters, though spiritually in the dark, were hardly 'at the Mill with slaves' or blind for that matter. A couple lie splayed out on a roof when the dog falls from the sky, splat. (I was less keen on the Marxism than on the upper-class twittery, which I thought sophisticated.)

Who reads Huxley now? As a teen-ager I loved him passionately. I fancied being a deracinated, intellectual Mrs Huxley, leading my spouse through canyons on a green string; I even made one of my lengthy voyage plans on how to get to California without paying, stowing on a boat and hanging under trains.

Failing that, to be Mrs Bertrand Russell.

Jane Austen wanted to be Mrs George Crabbe, and the critic George Saintsbury wanted to marry Elizabeth Bennet. How weird is that!

When she was 12 or so, Jane Austen wrote a story called 'The Beautiful Cassandra'. The heroine walks out of her mother's millinery shop, steals, hits, scoffs, ignores people and refuses to pay for a hackney cab; when she returns to her loving mother, she hugs her and remarks, 'That was a day well spent.' (More admirable than pert Lizzie Bennet with her sly pursuit of the best house, her scorn for girls who'd put in years of work on spoilt young Darcy.)

I now see one's better reading Jane Austen than Milton, Dylan Thomas, Huxley, Russell or Dostoevsky. With her in tow, I'd have arrived more completely at that rich, refined existence I once expected if only I read the right books and attended the right college. And more quickly if you compare her succinct little volumes with the great bloated monster of *Karamazov*.

The Beautiful Cassandra as role model (instead of drunken, sexy Grushenka)? Nothing cancerous and repressed about that girl.

If you *do* want a literary guide to get through ordinary life in 'the midland counties of England' – death too probably – then Jane Austen is for you. Courtesy not candour, good style (no loudness), self-restraint, some passion but no urge to *seek* unrequited and torturing love.

As for me, I stayed too long with the chaps and their gigantic, rambunctious emotions. They streamed through the firmament like never-ending fireworks to the music of Handel – or, worse, gloriously vicious Monteverdi. Then I tripped into unruly Mary Wollstonecraft, who hardly felt alive unless in turmoil: fusing for me struggle, risk and cruelly idealistic feminism. It's all contributed to an unquiet life.

On the couch, I peer again under my spectacles at the bare torso, the sad grey limbs. The machine doesn't reject me, I almost weep with gratitude. The poor bubbling skin takes the assault as LA8 cackles and trundles round, beeping and burping by Big-Sea Water. Names surge up and flop down into the fuzz and fur my mind's becoming.

'Everyman, I will go with thee, and be thy guide, in thy most need to go by thy side,' says Knowledge in those worthy little Everyman volumes. Yes indeedy, but is he there when dementia strikes and you go like sheet lightning?

Knowledge is science and science progresses. I'm here in Hospital-land with no 'transferrable skills', no Knowledge to speak of or listen to. Not even seeing through a glass darkly. (Father would be wondering who made that glass and how it got its tint.) My only 'knowledge' some drabs and dribs of Literature. They don't give much status here.

*

My brilliant friend N now demented out of all except pleasantries and scattered literary knowledge. Old, kind, warm, woolly Aunty with her moustache and large heart, removed from her house for setting fire to the sheets when smoking in bed; soon she knew neither right nor left nor which way out or in through the corridors of the Home she never wanted to enter; yet she greeted everyone: How nice to see you. How do you do. Unused to television, she thought its smart young people saw through the screen the broken old, huddling in their brightly lit lounge. Where's the mind that goes away, cracked and leaky as an old teacup? If it goes, who's left there? (Moments before her death, when we thought consciousness quite fled, Aunty reached out to put her finger on my lips.)

I wish I had a notion of medicine. Why did I drop Physics at 13? If I hadn't, could I have been walking the corridors in a white coat, my head stocked with pharmaceutical cant instead of Hiawatha and Fern Hill? Yesterday I had a Christmas card from a colleague of H's, another head of house: I have seen your scan – I am so sorry, it said. Yes, me too. Come join me in my low-residue diet for Christmas.

All those lives I might have lived.

A distant acquaintance has thrown herself in the river. She was serious when many pretend to seek death with pleading notes and too few pills. Something heroic there, taking the painful way. (Unable to lure Odysseus to the shore with her song, Parthenope drowned herself, her aesthetic failure too great.)

I'm sad and cross. If only I'd had her healthy flesh. When you're diseased, you think health is everything.

As I go through the hospital 'Hub', I see people in Costa Coffee eating nutty muffins and drinking strong coffee. A pledge-signer in a public house not more alien than I am. D would like a chocolate muffin but refrains out of pity.

My uncle suffered a stroke in his Baptist pulpit. Great aunts Myfanwy and Sarah went demented after years of caring for others; a grandfather was gassed to death. They didn't have cancer. It's not *obviously* genetic.

Live life to the full, people keep saying.

Full of what? Is it tasting everything on offer?

Offerings are not always mild. Nasty bits aren't improving.

'What doesn't kill you makes you stronger.' Well no, actually. Samuel Richardson's greatest heroine, the achingly virtuous Clarissa, fended off her aggressor for 6 long volumes, was raped, then remarked that her once fine temper was ruined.

Exactly. One isn't made stronger by misfortune, simply sourer.

Do you think Job just got over it after all that buffeting by God?

Oh to be healthy and half-fulfilled. Please.

Will I be blamed for being insufficiently positive? Will it be My Fault?

No need for unseemly detail, but all my big diseases have been noisy. Asthma and dysentery make a fine orchestra. Radio sickness too.

Oscar Wilde, that most sensitive of men, once he'd turned corpse in the dingy Parisian Hôtel d'Alsace, exploded in an unseemly mess of blood and bodily fluids. If one has to explode, best it be done in private in a house with a tolerant, kindly companion who's slightly deaf.

This morning I give myself an enema, so that between treatments I can be poked in yet another part. If you have 2 cancers and a recurrence, why not 4 and 5?

A sigmoidoscopy. 1 in 5000 perforate the bowel and from then onwards faeces must exit through a hole in the stomach. That's me, surely. (Before Cancer 2, a nervous lady with a stiletto probed the uterus and pierced it, so I had to wait 8 dragging weeks for healing.) 'I'm the sort of person an incontinent pigeon chooses to shit on,' I'd said when I heard. Nobody smiled.

This time the probe only travels part way. Am I perhaps not properly relaxed? Far enough, claims the doctor. I of course doubt, but thank him all the same: he's not pierced a vital organ.

I slide off his softer slab in what I intend as a jaunty way, but slip on the vinyl. Different floor surface from radio-onc, I remark, but he doesn't hear. He's on to the next patient and there's a room full of people with leaking bowels to peer into.

Now to Father in the Treatment Centre. I know my way along the Quentin Blake corridor and the space pictures, dragging myself up and down the stairs (virtuously instead of the lift) in Hospital-land where the ground outside must be ignored. Ground is nothing – you want level 2.

Just before I reach his bed, I meet Consultant X. He's with my friend H. I become an equal because she's my friend. I look grey, tired and shabby in my uneven red skirt. He ignores my state. As he should. 'If I were a betting man,' he says pleasantly, 'I would put a fiver on you.' He and H smile down at me benevolently, like indulgent parents.

After his always kindly greeting Father begins on what concerns him. I don't want to know. Nothing is firm anywhere, let's take that as read. I shut my ears. We whisper about his consultant, Miss G, who won't ring and speak to me and hardly has time for him either. Young, he says, from which I conclude 40s. Not gracious. I'm so sorry: he finds almost all women who aren't 'harridans' 'charming'.

So pathetic a sight. Usually dapper, his whispy white hair straggles along the pillow. He closes his real eye, the false one stays open. In the night he had an accident, never before in his life and so horrid, only hinted at, he pauses, so unlike him to pause. He cleaned himself up, put offending clothes in a plastic bag, and rang the bell. After much time a male nurse came and slapped new pyjamas on the bed. There was no smile or word of help or comfort, and he himself always so courteous.

'Perhaps he didn't speak English,' said Father, 'but he could have smiled.'

No one's paid enough for niceness. Friend S told me that, once on a plane to Washington, a very fat lady spilled into her seat. She tried to push back some of the encroaching flesh, so she could raise an arm to hold a book. 'Lady, you should have gone Business if you want to read,' said the fat woman. Perhaps you have to go Business to get a smile in the night.

Father so loves the kindness of strangers and he himself is kind to strangers. I am more uneasy, liking a smile indeed but not too much professional tenderness.

Father says he must live at least till August, the 100th birthday, and see Our Baby become one almost the same day. The baby with his name, the name of his grandfather, the itinerant ballad singer with his concertina in a wooden box.

I say I'd like to be there too.

20 December, Tuesday

LA8 is upset again. Its cooling system malfunctions. It needs a rest, says M. It wants its Christmas break. 'It fancies mince pies for a few days rather than human organs,' I say. M politely smiles.

A prostate and I are sent to LA5 where other silent people are waiting. I've bought the *Guardian* but can't face it. I notice a single

Country Life in the magazine pile. *Country Life* here? I used to look at pictures of posh houses in secret: middle-class porn to be ogled in Victorian replica bathrooms made from small third bedrooms. Not now. On a spare seat a discarded *Sun*.

The waiting men and one woman look askance at us coming on to LA5. Will it delay them? Will we take too many rays? No camaraderie here.

We're fitted haphazardly into the schedule and I'm on the slab with greater speed than usual, boots off in the corridor, then skirt in the passage, knickers down, heave up, splay out. There's a crooner on. Isn't the machine's purring and peeping enough?

Everyone in a hurry because we're too many. Feeling slightly more alert than usual, I find silly phrases floating around as I lie with the machine. Fanny Burney's 'shackles of fortuitous circumstances'. What use is that? Mary Wollstonecraft's envious sister Eliza wrote, 'I seem to take a pleasure in making those I love feel exactly the same degree of misery.' Wisdom there. Nice sometimes to know other people are wrecking their lives too, or having them wrecked. Nice being here with other people waiting to be hurt.

I finish my treatment. In come the protected girls, the machine goes quiet. Before my knickers are up, the next (male) patient arrives. I cover myself quickly, they bundle him out. 'Exit. Pursued by a Bear.' He apologises as I pass holding my boots and skirt. 'Hello,' I say. I have no particular shame for the part that's let me down.

Bowels, bladder, vagina – or what's left of the pelvic area, I've nothing to say to you, nothing, except Shape up, function properly and get a grip. Especially that: a good grip.

After elongated childbirth (unassisted production being in vogue in 1960s England), cystitis and bladder cancer, I tried pelvic exercises.

'You see women doing them at the bus stop,' said a nurse. 'You can do them anywhere.'

That withdrawn, meditative look females sometimes have doesn't mark a rich inner life, just fear of incontinence; not introspection but a poor bladder.

I go to the Treatment Centre to see Father. On the way I encounter H doing her sharp politeness in the corridor. Her boots have silver ornaments on a black base and are elevated by long spiky heels. There's a small discreet silvery zip. She negotiates the steps with ease. They'd be bad in a muddy field, I think. But they'll never go there: smart wellies for country walks. I love those boots – they shine with good health – I love scuttling along behind them in my flat pair with a protruding zip and leather bulge at the ankle. Trying to match her pace, responding to the cheeriness.

The bladder lures me on till I find myself in a new toilet complex. When I emerge, H has gone. Instead there's an old woman in a pink tracksuit and blond wig being pushed in a wheelchair. I arrive alone at level 5.

Father says there were whores in red and gold here last night entwining round curtain poles. His white strands of hair are blowing in the fan breeze from the next bed and the false eye looks fierce. He's high with his morphine drip I realise, but he doesn't know it. The first time I've ever seen him not in his right mind. His anger's real. He usually reserves it for MPs, union bosses, government interference, and overpaid GPs, but only when he doesn't know them.

He's explaining how the whores got in. His mode is always narrative. When you ask if he went to the doctor, he says, 'Well it was just after 11 and the sun was shining on the pub opposite and I looked in on the charming lady next door, whose son has just brought . . .' This will last out a winter night in Russia.

The old repeated war stories are marvellous, the Battle of Norway, the evacuation from St Nazaire, the battleship to Scapa Flow, the great fire at Cherbourg, the sinking of the *Lancastria* (Mother and I sceptical of this monstrous catastrophe which turned the sea into a black oil-pool of drowning men; Churchill hid the loss to keep up morale in a failing war – it became common knowledge only in our unheroic times), Montevideo, Mombasa, Alexandria, lying in the snow in a Greek ravine with a gun barrel at his forehead, the stolen jeep in Venice, the chess playing and unrationed dinners in New York, the iniquity of Lend-Lease and its leaky boats, the famous artist in Naples who swapped paintings for cheese – the lovely indistinct horse-scapes still on the walls of his flat – Father's own smelly cheese travelling from Milan to Wales and ponging the little train; then beyond the war the elephants and buffalo shoots and crazy games of men dressing as pantomime cows in jungle clearings and old imperial outposts, all manner of marvels when the world was quite different. Stories that clutch at the heart, my heart now I'm growing weak and sentimental.

Surely nothing will silence him.

The morphine wears down. Seamlessly he thanks us for coming.

21 December, Wednesday

For breakfast I push white bread into my dry mouth. Like eating a feather pillow or cotton pad. 'Bread of heaven' – we belted out 'Guide Me O Thou Great Redeemer' in school. 'Feed me till I want no more.'

In America I tried to persuade myself to like bean sprouts and sparkling water. An austere 1970s fashion of a country that didn't know much of forced austerity.

Neither allowed now: both make a great wind.

*

The proposed doughnut diet is – in essence – starch and sugar. Yet it's still not crystal clear. The Web says no bananas, the hospital says yes bananas but no tomatoes. The Web is silent on tomatoes. Is it to pleasure the machines we cut out so much? They don't want to burn windy bodies? Or is it to avoid constipation or diarrhoea? Can you have both? Yes, yes, I know the answer.

You can. So Merry Christmas.

No mince pies, no fruity Christmas cake, no plum pudding, no dates and figs, no gin and tonic, no red or white wine, no Brussels sprouts and cranberries. Merry Christmas.

Time to go out into the dark. A little spit of water in the air.

Fear is seeping in. Larkin's 'dread of dying and being dead'.

Be Positive. Fear is only the Sublime.

And the incipient darkness?

Nox perpetua, una dormienda. Darkness deepens. Embrace it. Or back to the battle, the combat.

Smother fear with white bread and Victoria sponge.

After the first cancer and before the second, a friend gave me a book about fighting disease by eating nuts and pulses. Now they're forbidden. Had I rejected the machine and embraced natural remedies like herbal teas, complex vitamins, deep breathing and emptying the mind, crystals or aromatherapy with golden scented lights cascading through me, acupuncture or meditation to serenity with New Age music, or developed my astral body, any- and everything except chemicals and manically editing books and moving house, would all have been well?

Or, if I'd crossed my fingers more firmly, glued them stuck?

Kept hold of the juju?

*

When it comes to it, will I now say, Bring on the morphine? Perhaps not, given Father's encounter with night whores. What unconscious might be revealed?

When D and I visit him today, he's back in his mind but his pain is palpable. We don't stay long. He closes his one eye. He must be very ill indeed, else he would be talking and saying how glad he is to see us. Over and over, enthusiasm being his mode.

As a college president I conferred Cambridge degrees in Latin in the Senate House, dressed in robes meant for men or stouter women. Unaware ahead of time I had to memorise *all* the Latin and that I had to parade, doffing the cap while holding on to the heavy furry stuff for fear of tripping, I didn't make the best job of it. But I was much moved to see each of our students so serious and happy in our awkward, intimate ceremony.

Less moved to spy Father sitting (enthusiastically) in the front row of the audience.

'How on earth did you get in?' I asked when I caught up with him later: the event was ticketed and limited to students' immediate family and friends.

'Ah,' he said, 'I stood by the door and told them I was an old man and had lost my ticket but I so very much wanted to see my daughter.' Assuming a student great-granddaughter, I suppose, they ushered the doddery old chap into the front row.

'Don't do it again,' I said.

When he came to Venice for his 95th birthday, C surprised him by flying in for just 2 nights from West Coast America: his delight flamed up like fireworks over the lagoon. Visiting the Hotel Danieli after 60 years was nothing to that (too quick for us, he noticed the prices on the menu: we had coffee and shared 2 buns).

*

At home I ring up a once-a-year-Christmas friend to tell her I'm on the third cancer. I sit back to await that comforting sympathy that brings a choke to the back of the throat. She says she has a spot of arthritis in her left foot and is planning to have Christmas with her stepbrother, then she laughs. If it doesn't involve imminent death, I really can't be doing with it.

I might be dying, I say dramatically.

We're all dying, she says.

Oh, I know that. But, actuarially, I'm likely to go before you. Look what I'd have to pay for medical insurance if I went to Florida. (I've been invited to lecture there and yearn to go from this dreary winter. I haven't cancelled yet.)

We exchange comments about the absurdity of Christmas cards.

You can't orchestrate sentiment.

In the late-afternoon dark, I struggle up the stairs to Father's flat to get some striped pyjamas which they probably won't let him wear. Only in the last months has it shown his age: a magnifying glass left on a chair, handrails by the toilet and shower. Nowhere he's lived alone has been quite as immaculate as the houses, flats and bungalows Mother kept as we rolled around the world, though he's tried to keep up standards by ironing tea-towels and underwear and always wiping the draining board dry. On the table I see his big black manual typewriter on which he wrote his impassioned formal letters of protest to newspapers, to HMRC on my behalf, and to the Council in gratitude for their flowerbeds or anger at their deplorable architecture. All with the slightly loose, much used ribbon. Next to the typewriter, his almost empty bottle of Tippex.

A folder of paper on his little desk: 'Instructions in case of death.'

They're prefaced by a heart-breaking note to me: 'You did not expect me to leave you on your own facing this, did you?' There follow details of what I should do to avoid paying for probate and for investment of any funds. All his life so careful with records and figures.

'No point in using a solicitor for something so simple, you can do this,' he writes.

Not without you.

How he'd like to have been a financier, a banker, or a stockbroker. Happier? Doubtful, he could not love a hyacinth more for all the world's riches. But he craved the education he's proud I've had. A curious, intelligent boy, he was offered the only scholarship at the Grammar, then a bursary for boys of war victims at the Duke of York School. His mother, with her widow's pension and 4 children, said she'd manage his un-earning years. But his teacher took him aside and told him he shouldn't add to her burdens. He doesn't forgive this long-dead man. (Mother was out of school at 14, while her brother went on to prepare for the ministry. Top of her class, she consoled herself by helping write his sermons, fostering a self-esteem she never lacked. Where Father wished he'd had education, Mother believed herself equal to those who had: that was enough.)

I wish I'd known Father more when I was growing up.

I go home slowly, taking in McDonald's in the town centre, out of my way but their facilities so welcoming. I hope they understand: I don't exist in a normal space and need humouring. Not disabled but not quite abled either. Certain organs – you know.

More Victoria sponge in the kitchen, really stale now. If I recover I won't eat another stale slice, even to be polite.

22 December, Thursday

The 12th session. Must study the Macmillan booklets. Plenty of time between the Shipping Forecast and 7.20.

Some of the long-term side-effects of radiotherapy can be the same as symptoms of cancer coming back. Just think of that, eh Hedda (as boring Tesman kept saying). Or LA8 turning against me: LA8, Preserver and Destroyer.

Over the page. Some women have to make changes to their life to accommodate the effects. Yes, yes, it would be as well to do so.

Thick knickers? No tight stylish trouser suits?

Not enough.

Changes can mean curtailing activities, less socialising, reducing or giving up work through need to stay close to a toilet.

Can't you talk through the bathroom door?

In Buñuel's *Phantom of Liberty*, the taboo is eating; defecating is social: so guests sit at table on toilets peeing and shitting from one end, but go into a private room to stuff sandwiches in at the other.

You can get a little card saying that you HAVE to use the nearest toilet.

Private homes? March up a garden path, flash your card like a search warrant, and demand access to the bathroom?

You can have a key that lets you into secret places in central squares, shopping arcades and railway stations.

Another section. Sexual effects. It may take longer to reach orgasm.

Can they be serious? Anything left down there to vibrate after these burning weeks? Are they confusing cancer with consumption? A burning, poetic, Keatsian desire supposedly afflicted the dying consumptive.

Sex was sometimes thought an antidote to consumption. Does it work for cancer?

The booklets are written by the well, and the groin, as Tristram Shandy remarked, is upon the very curtain of the place.

Less primly, Crazy Jane said, 'Love has pitched his mansion in / The place of excrement.'

Quite, said the Bishop, forcefully dismissing the 'foul sty'.

Lou Andreas-Salomé said the vagina is 'taken on lease' from the rectum.

Three orifices so near together, all opening and closing at their own sweet pace. It's no way to make a body. When the Lord cursed Eve for her sin with sorrowful birth, nothing was said of the follow-up.

Some people find they don't have much control of wind. Say that again.

William Blake's Nobodaddy farts and belches up there in his smelly heaven. Rabelais's giant Pantagruel had a fart that 'made the earth shake for twenty-nine miles around, and the foul air he blew out created more than fifty-three thousand tiny men, dwarves and creatures of weird shapes, and then he emitted a fat wet fart that turned into just as many tiny stooping women.' Misogyny, but there's the past for you. Edward de Vere of Aubrey's *Brief Lives*, bowing low to Queen Elizabeth, 'let a Fart, at which he was so abashed and ashamed that he went to Travell, 7 yeares. Upon his return, the Queen welcomed him home, and said, "My Lord, we had forgot the Fart."' (An oft-told, travelling tale, but none the worse for that.) No fart in Jane Austen's oeuvre, but, had she delivered one, it would surely have resembled the ladylike 'little fart' of Mrs Post in Elizabeth Taylor's elegant Home Counties' novel.

The booklet says many things make cancer more likely. Cigarettes. Poor diet. Too much alcohol. Obesity.

Why do they have it in for obesity? Why this trying to make fat people feel bad? I think of my long-ago flabby self.

Remembering when Black became Beautiful in the early 1960s and stayed so, making us whiteys feel that bit lacklustre. Why was there no Fat is Fine movement? Why such malevolence towards the obese? (I'm suspicious when public opinion and government agree.)

No need for smugness. I'm in the red band for osteoporosis. This comes in part – wait for it – because I'm thin. Cuddly people with fat on their shoulders are less vulnerable; bird-framed women, like Mother and me, when they fall, they break, not bounce. They shatter into 100 spiky pieces. And never really walk alone again.

Mother's brittle bones did for her: she couldn't face the shame of a Zimmer frame with its bustling little basket for shopping or knitting; so she sat, simply waiting.

By the end she'd had quite enough. She liked wifely dependency, always a social game. The physical sort was unappealing.

All the fun I refused, and look now. But then of course and finally: mostly, it's due to genes and chance. Yup to the second.

Fortune: Lakshmi, with her trickster's ingenuity.

Bitterly cold as we trundle through the car park, my breath steaming, the freezing air going up my bare thighs above the long socks. I mourn the Viyella trousers. Never a one for hip-hugging jeans, but I thought those trousers sleek and snug.

I pull the skirt round my legs against the wind, coldest it's been this year. 'The parching Air Burns frore, and cold performs *th' effect of Fire.*' Milton knew about burning cold.

Female skirts invented because of the curse, the flowers that stain, the bundling clouts; so why did old women have to wear them? Why not make it a proud mark of menopause to quit the skirt and don trousers (tight or loose depending on culture)? Like putting your hair up at menarche. A sign of achieving peace, solace, emotional emancipation.

In Ceylon, we assembled for what Father said was the wedding of his assistant's daughter. Bedecked in jewels, garlands and silk sari, the girl stood in an arch of flowers and paper festoons. Father jovially (and repeatedly) congratulated the bride and her parents and hoped the groom was just as handsome. It dawned first on Mother that we weren't celebrating a wedding but the girl's first period. Since I knew nothing of what was to come, the eventual understanding was lost on me. Now I think the ceremony a nice idea. No garlands and sweetmeats for menopause, even there.

LA8 doesn't like the cold. The big freeze last night upset it. The girls tell me it's not the newest machine. My loyalty is misplaced.

I go to LA1, the same square eye, the same hissing and beeping. The attendants scuttle off as usual and I'm left.
    Do I want Christmas music?
    I do not. Crooning carols and jazzed up plainsong, no, no.

Afterwards, I pull up loose knickers, my sad rump so abashed by the great eye. It can't protect itself and I can do nothing for it.
    Not even the starving would fancy these poor cuts of meat – not if I made them the most Modest Proposal.

Christmas is coming and the machines will be on what people now call 'annual leave'. When we return to Hospital-land, workers will have jettisoned their Santa hats and perky antlers.

The Bury couple are nearly finished. Soon I'll be the longest here, Mother of the Machines. Perhaps new patients will give me a coin or two when passing my chair, as they did Dickens's old Mr Dorrit when he became the longest inmate of the Marshalsea Prison.

Up to Father, who's looking grey and shrunken. He keeps patting down his unruly hair. Whenever he lifts his arm to calm it, he confuses the drips, feeds and tubes, making their controls chirp and squawk. He's not slept, nothing is staying down, neither end works. He's lower in spirits than usual and worse in body, his hairy chest rattling with infection despite antibiotics. And his bowels – well.

There wasn't anything wrong with his chest when he came in. What's happening?

He clutches at his *Telegraph* and manages a little comment on public sector pensions, but his heart's not in it. He looks at the crossword; it doesn't engross. No whisky, little indignation, no enthusiasm: he's becoming a shell of himself.

Yet, when, a few minutes later, C brings in her Baby, the frail old arms lift him high above the frail old cratered head, though he weighs like a sack of baking potatoes and the tubes beep alarmingly. The Baby chortles and wriggles his legs and as he comes down he puts his chubby hands in the old man's mouth and Father bites them playfully and the Baby smiles his toothless winning smile. And it is lovely. It is so happy days, says Father. He is a grand little fellow. And he is.

Hope for the best and prepare for the worst, he used to say. Accept what you can't change and change what you can, gain the wisdom to know the difference. He likes the common saying and refines it in different ways, but the gist always remains. Is he debating whether at last to try for acceptance? I doubt it. He'd never willingly leave life.

Will he recover or will he break in the sun as the sun breaks down, and death takes dominion? I don't know any more. As for me, Dylan's unicorn evils are already running me through. How can you be so tired and not be falling asleep or dead? Oh, Dylan, leave me be. Go off with Hiawatha paddling over Big-Sea water up the Towy estuary.

D and I go out of the hospital into the air to find the grass shining and iridescent in frost as never seen in near 70 years. Each blade a beauty and rebuke to living anywhere but Now.

*

I'm at home when Father rings to tells us he has *Clostridium difficile*. Caught in hospital. They tell him he's to go into a room by himself, and later to an isolation ward.

The Baby with his vast baby life and I in the middle of treatment . . .

I phone the ward to query selfishly about Us. A man answers. No, he says, no 4-month-old baby should have been in a colo-rectal or urology ward. Nor an elderly person on radiotherapy. Common sense.

Well bugger me! Thank you, I say. Thank you so much for telling me now.

I bargain with Lakshmi and the BVM, though they never keep their side. Do not let Our Baby be harmed; do not, and I will – what will I do? Build another cathedral in Venice and bury my sad torso in the foundations?

I feel better when, on the Web – the first time that's happened – I find *C.diff* hardly lives outside Hospital-land – except it might affect people on treatment or antibiotics. It doesn't seem to fancy babies. It will be All Right.

Christmas unfolds downstairs. D has dressed a tree with white lights and baubles, and put silvery parcels underneath. Pretty and sparkling. In the kitchen, rich food I can't eat and don't want.

Nothing sparkling and rich mounts to my attic bedroom with its lavatory in a cubicle. Not a modern ensuite but so welcome.

No one intrudes.

There are moments when being alone is what you want, but I appreciate good people on the ground floor.

*

In the first Christmas with real presents in warm Bermuda, I had a lavishly illustrated book meant for colonial children, *Our Island Story*, a warm and conceited history of England with anecdotes of conquest and victory and much bow-wowing about the Island Race. Mother gasped when she opened a box of black lingerie not seen outside a magazine. On a road in Upper Volta I missed Christmas, having no calendar, and never knew the lack; in Poland we queued for hours for sage, then paid millions of zlotties for some wilted leaves, we saw carp swimming in the neighbours' bath and ate cakes covered in poppy seeds, C and I mistaking them for chocolate chips; in the jolly Puerto Rican outdoors, babies sang, mine babbled in Spanish underneath the piñata.

Some time after the night-time Shipping Forecast and before the World Service's African digest, I'm in front of the Web, drawn in fly-like.

The current management of local recurrence after previous surgery is of limited efficacy. Successful salvage therapy can only be sought in patients with limited vaginal relapses. The overall 5-year survival rates measured from the time of recurrence ranged from 20% – 50%.

This is worse than the radiologist, brisk Dr Y, predicted: a lady of few pleasantries but good style.

I try to smile at the screen, but I can't humanise it. It's no LA8. In our series, the article continues, staring at me, the cure was only achieved in less than one-third of cases and the median survival after the diagnosis of recurrence was merely 20 months.

Now wait for the conclusion.

The efficacy of salvage radiotherapy in endometrial cancer patients with local failure after previous surgery is limited. Factors determining treatment outcome include advancement of the tumour at relapse and radiotherapy dose.

*

Limited. Limited. A liminal space. A panicking space. Twisted to my purpose (I know, I know).

I should have ingested Jane Austen properly. I was no better than Catherine Morland: after making a complete goose of herself before her betters, she understood that all she experienced had been 'forced to bend to one purpose by a mind which . . . had been craving to be frightened.'

But, as with my worthy teen-age extracts, *Northanger Abbey* gives its stern advice too late.

I send an anguished message to friend S in America.

She emails back: there should be parental control software to block you from these sites.

I've thought of Father's funeral. Mobilising the British Legion with their flags, banners and brass band – he spoke with pride of his own father's send-off with 'The Last Post' played by 2 buglers over the flag-draped coffin. But then he said he'd rather like the humming chorus from *Madame Butterfly* at the crematorium; not sure that can be done with a British Legion band. I'll invite the patrons of the cosy pub who bring in flowers and sadly inedible food, the wonderful publican with whom he exchanges good cheer and quips – 'Such a lovely lady,' he always adds when mentioning her, such good beer there, so snug in the corner surrounded by his little court.

Who will reach the grave first? Him or me? Has he been planning *my* funeral? I'd like the end of Schubert's Quintet, just the end, and perhaps a Dylan reading?

I mean *Dylan* reading, in that lugubrious, artificial voice of his.

*

Father remembers how, in his choirboy years, the high cross stuck in his cassock as he paraded it down the aisle; he had to lift it so high the congregation thought he saw a vision or had run mad. Now, in old age, he's become an atheist. Yet he wants to hear, well have others hear, Those Words, dust to dust, ashes to ashes, for man born of woman, and so forth. The 'lovely' publican is also a Christian minister. Would she say those words – and forget the Resurrection? Too much to ask, but I will, if it comes to it.

One last thing: he doesn't want that dirge of a hymn they can never resist in Wales: 'The day thou gavest, Lord, is ended, The darkness falls at thy behest.'

In Puerto Rico, lacking suitable books and lost without something to research, a friend and I ransacked our minds for what we'd stored there. We found hymns. So, we wrote of their creation in the 18th century, discovering their theatricality – singers acting out little, apocalyptic scenes of fear and salvation right there in open fields or bare wood chapels. The pre-eminent hymn of my part of the book was John Newton's 'Amazing Grace'; sadly 'Guide me, O' was originally in Welsh, so not included. (Mother heard somewhere she might be related to its author, William Williams of Pantycelin: no means of knowing, since genealogy with a name like 'Jones' is challenging.)

It struck me then how demanding these hymns were. Telling the deity to guide, feed, hide, lead, succour, cleave rocks. It isn't quite John Donne's insistence that God ravish him to make him chaste, but the demands are pretty peremptory, considering the addressee.

The dust and ashes Father so liked from the Book of Common Prayer exist for me too on the thin paper of the ivory-backed copy I received at my confirmation in school. The North Wales Baptist chapel was Welsh-speaking; otherwise I might have had immersion in a nearby river – way more dramatic. (As it was for deaf Aunty, who stopped being completely deaf after this dipping. It happened during a prayer meeting held on a cold spring day. She heard birdsong for the first time.)

Instead, I was saved from the 'devil and all his works' by the portly Bishop of St David's amply filling the episcopal seat for the Bishop of St Asaph's. He was indisposed, so never saw me for the first time in court shoes and nylon stockings renounce the 'sinful lusts of the flesh'.

If only they'd been on offer. But if there were boys anywhere I didn't see them and we girls were so policed we weren't even to sleep in beds next to friends or sit together for meals. My grown-up self assumes the headmistress repressed a lesbian inclination and knew what she was about with this panoptical surveillance. At the time, I thought it just another prop of Discipline.

The fat prelate did me some service. How it was I can't tell, but my apostasy began at confirmation. Almost at once I felt such relief that the Lord was no longer in my head, seeing Every Nasty Thought. (In fact, I learnt, over many years, you can't rid yourself of him just by refusing to believe.)

My old prayer book was the red leatherette one given to pupils in Council School to celebrate the Coronation – Mother saw I got one though I'd been there so short a time. (She was usually a force when it came to inserting me into and taking me out of irritated schools.)

Received just before we flew up and away from London in June. We looked down on a wet, cold city emblazoned with fireworks. Perilously hopping over several days to Rome, Cairo, Basra, Karachi, Bombay and Colombo on the type of plane that fell out of the air so often – comet or constellation? – that Father tanked up in sizzling Karachi, worried, I now see, that we'd never make it to his next posting. Unaware of the peril, I was shocked when he paid 5 shillings for a beer. The price of an Enid Blyton *Famous Five* book – not perhaps in Karachi, but still. A drink instead of a book – my outrage was loud.

The next year I was to hold the Coronation prayer book as Mary in a Nativity play. Mother said I was chosen because of my long dark hair – to dispel any notion it was due to my mild character. Joseph would be Rodney, who shared a desk with me in school. Then came polio and in a week the little boy was dead. In England, the disease tended to maim and cripple, but in this steamy place it killed. The Nativity play was cancelled.

Father wants his ashes – when convenient, he hates being a nuisance – inserted into the churchyard in Mid-Wales. Mother went there but only after hers had lain for months in a pot in the wardrobe – the gracelessness of it! Foot and mouth restrictions forbade walking the path through the long grass beside the hawthorn bushes.

Foot and mouth indeed, said Father, pooh-poohing the national panic, Government Interference, cows shouldn't be fed on sheep, leave them chewing grass and they'd get better. When I was a boy . . .

A stately woman though under 5 feet in flat shoes, Mother would have hated the indignity of that top compartment in a *fitted* wardrobe. Ruining her solemn translation.

I was cross too, in an urban-rambler sort of way. Shouldn't we be able to walk on rural paths? Do carnivorous cows own the countryside?

23 December, Friday

To LA8. A portly, ponchoed, middle-aged lady, dyed black glossy hair, eyes startled by liner and mascara; she thanks the attendants again and again. Is this a good idea? Does it help? Does it ingratiate? Is this the right tone? Or is there a sly mocking expression in their eyes? Do I worry too much about tone? But it could be life and death in Hospital-land where patients should be courteous and cautious. (I recall my unappreciated remark about the shitting pigeon.)

*

As she passes me, I avoid the pained panda eyes in their black haloes.

My mind's blanked by salvage and ashes and the rogue bacterium, so that even the Hawk on Fire and Big-Sea Water can't enter today. I lie in the usual discomfort under the eye till the machine finishes its journey and halts. Eliot's duo of 'fire and the rose' in his *Four Quartets* are never One in here. Purgation and divine love? Purgation and pain under the icy sun?

Still on the couch, I mention the faintest possibility of *Clostridium difficile*. A hypothetical case. The girls stiffen. We would need to fumigate and stop treatment at once, it mustn't spread. I stiffen in turn and roll off in silence.

'Have a nice holiday,' they say, as I pull up knickers and hitch up skirt and answer, I hope cheerily, before dashing to the lavatory. 'Enjoy Christmas.'

For once, D's in low spirits. And why not? *His* cells aren't misbehaving and yet here he sits day after day in the bright light of Emmeline with only his Kindle for company. He'd never say so, but sometimes surely he must think this a bit unfair.

We walk out past the bicycle poem to the Hub. Where do consultants eat? Do they have poems in big letters and bright coloured art on their walls, a diet of Costa buns and Burger King burgers? Or do they drink superior coffee and eat Bahlsen biscuits in a tasteful, ecru-painted room?

No need for bitterness, I chide myself. Think instead of those lovely intricate postcards S sends almost every week from America of flowers and trees, of Mount Vernon and Monticello, of stark Bacon's Castle, visited when I worked on Aphra Behn and her play about the American rebel. Aphra writing when – as S tactfully fails to mention – extremely close to death. She didn't live to see her play performed. Just as well since it flopped.

Aphra, the most flaming of English women, the first to earn her own living – even more, the first to know no boundaries till banged against them.

Up to Father. Intercepted on the way by a nurse who says we can take him home for Christmas. Just for a few hours.

But he's not well is he, and his chest and bowels are bad; he can't – well how to put it? – and he hasn't even eaten the Weetabix which has turned to mush just out of his reach. And the *C.diff*?

'It's up to you,' she says.

'Well, no,' I say, 'it's not.'

Later Someone More Important says he cannot go out, even for a few hours.

Guilty that I didn't jump at the chance to take him home.

We reach him. I think again he's dead. But he rouses himself, his real eye concentrating as the plastic one stares fixedly elsewhere. By the end of the visit he's his garrulous, affirming self, reminiscing about Hot Cross buns nailed annually to the pastry-shop wall when he was a boy and telling us of the cleaner he's just met who makes mince pies to sell for charity.

Could he actually be on the mend? He's looking in the *Telegraph* – they don't take the *Guardian* at Sandringham he says. GPs earn £120,000 before overtime and they won't do weekends and evenings. Spoilt. In my day . . . he must be on the mend. We try to avoid the symptom-litany.

*

I get home just in time. Glued to the plastic seat in my little cubicle well into the night, rising every 10 minutes or so to flush and return. It's become a cucking-stool.

Into Christmas Eve as black comedy. Is this my worst day/night? If the bladder, bowels and guts hadn't become so demanding, the pain of getting out of the duvet would keep me rolled up in foetal pose.

Imagining a house 'where all's accustomed, ceremonious'. The male arrogance of Yeats's great 'Prayer for my Daughter' used to irritate: now its seductive rural serenity washes over me without my quite remembering the words.

Imagining, too, a fresh winded privy over a stream.

Best not pollute the winds and water.

In West Ireland, staying with friends in a hunting lodge, I had stomach pains and runs. Sitting in my ensuite, I heard other 'guests' in similar plight. Management insisted it was just me, then just consumers of bottled water, then drinkers of any water, then the fault of Sligo, then . . .

Like doctors or plumbers, hoteliers never apologise for what they cause.

I lean luxuriously on the radiator, grateful for this warm toilet in a cupboard, nowhere so cosy.

Tears come to my eyes and spill out quietly. I'm not constipated. How good is that? Always constipated in school and at Aunty's because so cold, too cold to wait long on the wooden seat. Too cold to use the newspaper cut up in squares and dangling on a string. Newspaper bits that enticed with their fragmented stories.

I have this in common with Father: I always want to know the rest.

Too many defecatory memories.

There's more.

Nkrumah Africanised production of toilet paper in Ghana: short-ages followed. British expats used the crinkly overseas *Guardian*s; newsprint stained anus and buttocks.

Working outside Delhi, I had a square bar of soap and a jug to catch water in the early hours.

Those scorching months teaching in Delhi and Jaipur. The horror of going with brave women to protest a sati of an 18-year-old girl in Deorala, drugged as like as not, but who's to say? The baying of young city men for the appalling sacrifice. You're white, you stick out, you'd better go, it's turning ugly, said my friends. I left through the streaming eager crowds. Something you don't forget.

Then down to C.D. Narasimhaiah's sweltering compound, Dhvanyaloka, Mysore. The squashed mosquitoes on the net, the swooshing of coconut palms, a meeting with the great R.K.Narayan (though CDN preferred talking to me of Dr Leavis – 'Why is his house in Bulstrode Gardens not a museum?'). My lecture on literary theory interrupted by an elderly man crying out, 'It's all in the Vedas.' The theft of all my documents and money just when the British consulate had gone on holiday. Finally, in desperation ringing my friend Anita Desai in America who'd arranged it all. Help, I said, before the line went dead, as it so often did.

Stress can cause cancer, says an article in the *Telegraph*. It does in fruit flies.

What stress do fruit flies have? Do they suffer from bullies, a poor temperament, a propensity to worry at 4 in the morning?

Pesticides, additives, meat, cooked and uncooked: so much causes cancer it's difficult to find your own special cause. It's a wonder any one of us is alive. Life causes cancer, life causes death, death stops cancer.

If you're properly cremated.

I'm circling on the pin of the point: giving credence where it's no business to be — those fruit flies — to *stress and cancer*. (Rage, unre-pressed, uncompressed?) 'The link is weak' but some find it 'clear'. If it *is* there, then wasn't Dotheboys Hall enough?

Not to sabotage a life.

In *Crime and Punishment*, a book read so often when I was a sucker for electrically charged Russian habits, Raskolnikov dreams he watches a horse beaten to death. I remember eating my own dog and cat in Ghana. Fattened up through a summer with money left for their care, then cooked by Kwesi in the stew to welcome my return. My fault: I should have clarified what was pet and what food. (In truth, difficult to tell with the cat — unlike an English beast that puts its tail straight in the air stalking round a city flat, more a scrawny hunter adopting me for scraps, not fondling.) I didn't see their slaughter and didn't vomit when I heard the stew's ingredients. But I was sad. Was this my Raskolnikov horse-beating moment?

What else might I have done? Is my type of self-deprecation too vain? Should I do guilt? More shame? Even remorse? Though that's fallen from fashion. Is guilt stress?

How about that divorce when I lost Everything. ('Only things,' Father said, gently, when we got back from New Jersey to Wales, and I told him his money was gone as well as my earnings. They only ever existed in America. But he cried for me as I'd never seen him cry for himself.) Revenge served neither hot nor cold: did this fester and grow cells in me? Is this the second source after Dotheboys Hall — overtopping that beastly stew? Norman Mailer said that, if he'd not stabbed his wife, he'd have got cancer and died. (Apparently, she provoked him by saying he wasn't as good as Dostoevsky.)

Everyone who's been divorced owns a divorce story, has run the gamut of furious cliché, has had to bottle rage. Mine lasted over 4 years and was bad. But 'Only Things'. Fragile things.

Besides, though he became monstrous to me, my fault was first: those constant illnesses, my intolerance of his failures – both would madden any husband. Sadly, as he persecuted me, I came to miss his obtuse, rigid but once gentle self, eventually remembering the long-ago dancing in sweaty, syncopated African air. A temperamental fault, a residue of that pre-feminist world I grew up in, which decreed that men should provide and dominate and, perhaps, be fierce? (Little of Father in this, but he was absent when ideas were shaped.)

I no longer regret the marriage ending, though I regret the whimsical, selfish cruelty visited on children while adults tussled. The courts, police stations and probation offices, the turmoil in the snowy bus station as state troopers flashed lights and roared, the dash to England on the rusting Air India plane before the American judge could enforce his order on American soil.

A dredgy, *ambiguous* memory – for what, in the end, was this escape but drama and another journey.

Blame the parents, blame the rebellious trend of the times.

Relieved to see my stoic boy and girl lay it all aside with grace.

I could go on. There's always more. Much more.

But, in the end, surely it's cancer that causes stress. Not the reverse.

My colleagues have given me a plant with little white flowers and a friendly message on it. I'm so grateful I overwater it and loose earth spills on to the table.

At least I can hold my own basin and close the door. I can still be secretive and (just a little) independent.

Care doesn't have to mean company and comforting words – it can come with tact, unlimited paper products and carafes of fresh water.

Christmas

I used to wonder what Christmas would be like without a talking father or a critical mother. I know now: not good. Not even with the delicious Baby banging away on his new toys.

We had no heart for celebrating. No one put on paper hats or read the dreadful jokes from crackers or listened to the Queen or Nine Lessons and Carols from Kings, or set the table just so and ate when everything was exactly 'piping hot'.

We thought we resented these things but we did them for him and her and then felt better that we'd done everything decently. A proper togetherness. So much we missed Father and his rituals and bonhomie, his appreciation of every titbit. Of everything about us.

We visualised him so strenuously that sometimes it seemed he was there, sitting on the sofa reading his Christmas books. We always gave him a single malt Glenmorangie – kept in the bedroom for drinking and sharing only with guests who knew better than to adulterate fine spirits with ginger or soda – books about the war or travelling in the 1930s. Without Mother's guidance, he gave us things advertised in the *Telegraph*: colourful pashminas and long scarves in cellophane packets, silvery necklaces, gift boxes of regional Italian olive oils and CDs of famous orchestras. All wrapped neatly in patterned paper often saved and smoothed out from the last Christmas. Everyone got a snowy card, bought to Help the Homeless.

In fact, I sat much of Christmas Day in my warm cubicle, while kind D and sweet C cooked and washed up.

I'm suffused by their goodness. How could I spoil my perhaps few weeks/months with nostalgia for pain, for a long defunct school, for grotesque American justice, when I have such good people down there in the kitchen? My brain as addled as my bowels.

Have the linings of both gone to mush? 'Buck up,' I say again, socks up. After all, Consultant X would put a fiver on me. (I could have wished a larger sum.)

No break from Hospital-land of course – we visited the Treatment Centre every day, bringing gifts of food and drink neither Father nor I wanted or could eat. His backside sore now as well as all the inner parts. He's marooned here in this leakiest of vessels. After going down with so many frigates and destroyers and always popping up in good if chastened spirits, is this his body's final sinking?

The television-cum-radio-cum-telephone intrudes but is beyond him or me – the radio is apparently free. I picked up its phone. A voice told me to put in my credit card. He just wants the radio, I said into its mouthpiece. Only one eye and it's not so clear, no point in television. 'Put in your credit card,' said the voice. I explained about the radio again. 'Put in your credit card.'

Mother too, before dying, spurned this contraption though we urged it on her.

Look, we said, this lets you phone and listen to the radio and watch television. You swing round the arm.

'I don't talk to the television,' said Mother, her gnarled fingers grabbing at the blanket, the plastic hospital label swinging large like an expensive bracelet. She knows Father has talked back when the news was too provoking or the Welsh were losing at rugby.

'You like the wireless, you know you do. You like Jenni Murray.'

And Mother, not demented but not in her right mind at this morphine-sodden juncture, said, 'She's no better than she should be.'

'She's on *Woman's Hour*,' I said, 'on the radio.'

'Oh, I dare say,' said Mother. Then she pursed her lips in the way she always did when disapproving, but the lips grew slack almost at once. Perhaps the spurt of disapproval gave a semblance of control.

She'd no objection to dying, but a horror of an open casket. We assured her the coffin, once occupied, would be promptly nailed down.

Next day Father seemed better in spirits. The Duke of Edinburgh had just left hospital with carloads of security guards and cameras. 'We served on the same ship,' said Father again, 'but on different decks.' He chuckled.

One winter morning in King's Lynn, in his 90s, Father marched out with his rows of medals pinned to his blazer and his black beret on the side of his head, as the Duke came to inspect the British Legion. HRH kept them waiting too long in the chilly air, then stepped from a heated car to shake a few hands. 'I remember the ship,' said the Duke to Father. He left them all so grateful. (I came to watch and of course caught cold.)

Father was never shy with Royalty. When I met him and Mother in Paris during my au pair year – shocking them with my dramatic change in shape, they being as ignorant of au pairs in France as of British boarding schools – we took a train to Versailles. Father spied the Duke of Windsor whom he admired for his much-touted remark about the misery of South Wales miners, that 'something should be done'. To my horror, he marched up to the ex-King and shook his hand.

Conversation followed and we were dragged over for introductions. HRH soon being at a loss, Father terminated the encounter by wishing him a long and happy life with his wife.

'Really!' exclaimed Mother, who didn't care for this ex-playboy, even less for Wallis Simpson.

Yet she too was seducible by the Royal or nearly Royal, commenting on the becoming 'informality' of Lady Mountbatten when they were women together over teacups in Ceylon. Discounting that wild love triangle of Mountbattens and Pandit Nehru – as Father discounted the Windsors' Nazi flirting.

How Royalty shadows our lives, year in, year out: it happened the year the King died, we say, the Queen married, bore child after expensive child. Chances are you die in a hospital graced with a royal name, the Princess Royal, the Queen Elizabeth, the Royal Alexandra. Can I go out in the Wollstonecraft Infirmary? Better still, in the Aphra Behn Rest Home.

In the meantime, no escape. Royalty always has something up its sleeve for a grateful nation, some entertaining scandal, some birth, marriage or long-awaited death.

The College was grateful when the Duke came to visit, making his usual gaffes. Amusing now he was so old – though dreadful when younger. I pointed out that many of our students had taken earlier degrees. 'Ah,' he said 'retreads.' He advanced towards a group of smiling Koreans, remarking, 'You're retreads I hear.' Bewildered, they yet shared the pleasure that he'd come and been so affable. (Royalty doesn't need to do much to be liked.)

My private Duke moment was in the Library lift: to make conversation I told him I'd given a radio talk about the Garden of Eden – i.e. Eden's Garden – in Venice, owned once by the Greek princesses Aspasia and her daughter Alexandra. 'Alexandra was a most beautiful woman,' he said with a rather faraway look – I think. I couldn't be sure, the lift being small and the Duke tall.

I tell Father the story again – a cheering little gift.

28 December, Wednesday

Back to Gormenghast in the early morning dark. The building looking dingier, the décor mustier. Even the artificial trees are wilting. I'm going down the wrong corridor while D jerks the car round and round the multi-storey park – or there's new art on the wall. Alice not more disoriented in Wonderland or Kafka in the Office. A man limps along in soft shoes on the arm of a stout lined woman with a glittering Santa Claus brooch on her lapel. She delicately holds the man's other hand.

I retrace my steps and finally ask. Like enquiring the way in the back *calles* of Venice. '*Sempre dritto*' and you know there'll be bridges and curves and false endings ahead, but at least someone must have recognised the reality of your destination.

I finally arrive at Radio-onc. The interval has made us all unreal. Waves of numbness roll over. Is there a bell jar above the waiting-room? One or 2 of us ask after Christmas and reply with a little recap of symptoms, but most are too tired to say much. A subtle collective consciousness of anxiety, of different degrees of acceptance and resentment.

Someone in the adjoining waiting area, maybe a novice, or yet undiagnosed, or with only 7 days of treatment, is telling with minuteness of his Christmas trip to Thailand using a wheelchair.

I look down at my rumpled skirt. Do not, I want to say, think that in my ordinary working life I looked quite like this. I'm not always this caricature, this weird elderly person dressed as a peasant girl in clashing colours. Never fashionable, but never this apology for a tramp. No matter. No one's looking, no audience after 60 . . .

I once said Good morning to the next client of LA8. He looked at me blankly. I was clutching my boots and brown scarf. Did he think I was mad or contagious? Should victims just keep their distance? Badinage only with the girls?

I'm called. LA8 must be rested, the growling and wheezing are a purr today. The seasonal music gone. Christmas as abruptly over in Hospital-land as outside. It used to linger at least to New Year if not quite to Twelfth Night, but now there's nothing but holiday brochures.

A wailing female voice sails over the machines. From the '80s or '70s? Real or retro the same to me. Is the orange new or the 1960s come back? It was always bilious. An acquaintance in Florida loved it so much her whole house was orange, from walls to toothbrush and dishcloths, clothes and lipstick. Something about the era that prevented you from asking Why?

Up on the carbon fibre with today a little modesty paper over part of the diminished pelvis (the cold ventilator whips it off). The big square-eyed machine wheels itself into place and its handmaidens bow out of the room leaving us again alone.

By the shores of Gitche Gumee.

Please no.

I try to recall something noble from Saint Jane. Nigel Nicolson being read *Pride and Prejudice* as he lay dying. Had I a choice at such extremity, I'd settle for *Mansfield Park*. Imagination quails at 'the thought of a Saturday night at the Edmund Bertrams, after the prayer-books have been put away', wrote mischievous Kingsley Amis. No 'quailing' necessary, for the acerbic author would be present – she always is in this masterpiece. But I'd dread teatime with the insuffer-ably smug Fitzwilliam Darcys – instead, give me cocktails with Lady Catherine de Burgh by the OTT fireplace.

Even with these thoughts, no Austen appears. I'm stuck in poetry: by the shores of GG and on Sir John's elmed hill. Suddenly I hear a mistressly RP voice reading 'Crossing the Bar' on the Home Service. 'Sunset and evening star, And one clear call for me!' Tally-ho.

New year soon, but tactless to wish it 'happy'. If said cheerily, it might seem over-exuberant. Or ironic. Never do irony round medical people and patients.

Fatigue is common. The tiredness may last for weeks or months after treatment. It can sometimes go on for a year or 2 in extreme form. So says the booklet. That is, if you are alive. What's fatigue compared with . . . ?

*

I note, that, whether or not tiredness diminishes, it's already marched off with a fair bit of me. I was always (inadvertently) a risk-taker, stepping first on the shaky bridge, diving into shallow water, crossing into Dahomey after my passport was filched, accepting jobs when warned of viperous colleagues, shacking up with the dangerous and disastrous, finding and holding the renegade idea. It isn't the best characteristic but it was a large part of me. I'm reduced: I no longer love risk or seek a place of fear.

Must wait for a new schedule. Gitche Gumee and the Great Grey Green Greasy Limpopo River circle on a loop. Tomorrow and tomorrow and tomorrow and tomorrow. Such tiredness, I lay my head against the wall; the top of the seat digs into my neck.

The Bury man said his review went well: he would live to a great age. Sceptic by nature – and envious, for no one has said anything like this to me———I query it but he's sure.

I ask the girls if it could be so – perhaps it's a man thing and the male privates are more susceptible to diagnosis. But no. None of us will know yet, they tell me. His joy is false. None the worse for that.

All over Christmastime I've adhered to the diet, eating only so much of parsnips and abjuring cabbage and sprouts, peas and beans. Sweet potatoes are on the prescribed list, but I thought it must be a mistake. I had a little with a pat of butter. The evidence is in the guts, no argument with them – or the bowels.

I curse the sweet potato which is no potato.

29 December, Thursday

A night in the cubicle with the radio on the floor. Imodium can't attack this. It's beyond pills. I'm still there when *Farming Today* comes on at 5.45 and repeats an earlier story about geese and turkeys. The rich had boars' heads, the poor caught little birds. I know that. Haven't I grown up on Father's rook pie and the Great Goose? Poverty and edible birds. The radio's tormenting. No wonder Father abandoned it unheard. Lost in his own programmes – a whole century to choose from.

I have no time for bed even in foetal position. Radios and radio-therapies are intermingling.

In too early to Emmeline, the contrast of dark outside and too bright clinical light within is jarring. Bury people up for review today, so not here. I miss their quiet hopefulness.

LA8 is being checked; I'm moved to LA1.

I hope the girls have forgotten I told them of *C.difficile*. The reaction was discouraging. I'm ashamed of my selfishness, but there it is . . . nothing so likely as disease to bring you face to face with your own shoddy egoism.

They don't mention the matter. I try to be affable. 'Attitudes are nothing, madam – 'tis the transition from one attitude to another which is all in all.'

Lying on the couch, crotch displayed, eyes wide open with sleeplessness, humiliation quietened, I can't help noticing that LA1 is shabby. Its paintwork needs renewing, its edges look frayed. Wouldn't be surprised to spy graffiti on its underbelly. I make out only a couple of letters with my short-sighted eyes, a few numbers scribbled in no very professional manner. It's not a loved machine.

I gaze into its wires and plugs above the square eye. Why on view? Other machines aren't so immodest. Does it make an ethical point? This is the real thing, surface polish of no account, the Wizard of Oz behind the curtain? The wired and tubed heart on show?

Me too. You old, scrawny, flabby bag of tubes and wiring gone wrong. If bladder and bowels and uterus et al. had had proper servicing once a week over the years (by professionals), would you now be in this breakdown room? Will there be another year on the road for you, or the scrapyard? I look down at it, softly.

We visit Father. He's so ashamed of his weakness he can't keep off the topic. Both of us so self-centred and talkative, as concerned with our produce as a toddler.

I worry he won't make his century. He so wants to be 100, 105. And I want it so much too. To have his royal telegram filched by death, all that life gone poof.

I think of him in kaleidoscope: his own pa gassed in the trenches of the First War and he valiant and cheerful through the Second, left with memories of dead bodies bobbing up through oily seas while he reached out to them with a wooden pole, passing up shells to gunners, kept down deep in the ship's hold as torpedoes gashed the side and bilge rose, going down in ship after ship, pulling on ropes with dangling icicles in the Arctic. But having young-men high jinks as Widow Twanky and Lady Bracknell in am-drams on shore in New York, Montevideo and Naples, hearing Tito Gobbi sing for a bottle of whisky.

Bringing home finally to Wales in 1946 a gilded angel's wing from Monte Cassino; a baroquely bound volume of Marcus Aurelius, the name a blank to him but reverenced for its mystery and gold lettering and, by the end, its comfortable sayings: 'If it is not right, do not do it, if it is not true, do not say it'; a Florentine china doll with come-hither eyes and lashes, called Annabel, bartered for with all he had once he knew himself father to a girl-child far away; and a tray of iridescent butterfly wings from India; small carved ivory elephants holding each other's tails.

What will happen to all these things when the twice-told tales, their aura, fade away? When he and I are gone?

One day, soon, no one will have memories like his.

*

Back in the house, just about to read a new cancer book which someone has pressed upon me with the best intentions . . . a phone call from Father. He says Miss G has come round the ward and said he will go home on Friday. Well now. He's indestructible. But he's also ill. He knows he is. We know it. What about the *C.Difficile*, the isolation? All forgotten.

He asked Miss G to phone me to explain but she doesn't. Has she looked in his file? Is there anyone out there? Care in the community is an elderly daughter in the midst of radiotherapy and a grand-daughter with a new baby. He won't want much Care: happier helping than being helped. But the pain and problems? How will he cope?

30 December, Friday

I'm on the computer at 4.30 a.m. 'Is there anybody there?' said the Traveller, / Knocking on the moonlit door.' No one awake, no friend to phone at such an hour. Only the entangling Web left— 'Keep off,' advises D, but he's asleep too.

I find Washington University School of Medicine. American. It must be good: look what they spend on healthcare. The article is about people like me treated with radiotherapy, full of percentages and words in red. All patients who had Grade 3 disease were dead by 3.6 years from the time of recurrence. That's not me – or is it after waiting through that long, hot, dropsical summer?

The starkness is exciting, none of this gyny-onc-optimism here. Do they think we don't read?

Off I go again, finding the survival rates after vaginal relapses – after salvage radiotherapy – have been reported in the literature to range between 25% and 68%. (I relish this savage word, 'salvage'.) A previous report concluded that patients who had extra-vaginal disease couldn't be salvaged with radiotherapy alone. They are excluded from this analysis. That is, they are dead. Those dead are excluded.

Early diagnosis, the repeated phrase – coals on the head of you, Consultant X and Miss G. Early diagnosis. Told you so. Right, so dead: I and poor old Father.

'Wretches hang that Jury-men may Dine.'

I'm being unfair, but I can't stop. It's still not morning enough for anyone else to be on a talking line or in Emmeline's waiting area. No one to stop me muddling words and numbers, clutching leading or misleading percentages, and blaming the (just) possibly blameless.

Isolated vaginal recurrences are rare; usually they are an indication of an underlying deep pelvic disease, which carries a poor prognosis. That's me. 10 years of yoga and pelvic twists counting for nothing.

I breathe slowly in through the nose and out through the mouth in thoracic gusts. Then plough on.

In 34% of cases the disease was extended to the pelvic wall. Progressing endometrial carcinoma was the cause of death in 16 of 29 stage I patients and in 22 of 25 stage III patients.

This is real, actuarial, these are figures worth writing down. 5-year disease-specific survival rates for stages I, II, and III: 86%, 38%, and 13%, respectively. From 86% to 38%! (The bravado of these medical men! Putting out papers as if commenting on Virgil.)

I must redo my will, move money into current account for easy payment of funeral expenses following hospice. Do I hear myself? Is this bravado? Is this garbled actuarial fluster a teeny bit theatrical? (Father has quietly, undramatically, prepared for after-death.)

In the *Guardian* I reviewed a fat panicking book by Joyce Carol Oates about her husband's death. Pages contemplating suicide and grumbling at too many gifts of fancy food and flowers from famous people. Turns out that, even before publication, she'd found a new mate and was very happy, planning to go exotic travelling. In the end, other people's misery, death is – well it's other people's; however close, however beloved, however much you'd change places, give up your life etc., you know you can't and haven't. You can recover from someone else's, as evidently Miss Oates did. Less easy with your own, eh? 'I never knew any man who could not bear another's misfortunes perfectly like a Christian.' Johnson? Pope?

Swift imagined friends contemplating his descent towards death: they 'hug themselves, and reason thus: "It is not yet so bad with us."'

Under the machine again. I know what it's about, I know how it will stop and start and go round and back. The haunts of coot and hern are there, Hiawatha and polly wolly doodle and hey nonny nonny all down the corridors, pit patting on wobbly puddleduck feet.

I want to sneeze and break wind, but everything must stay in. Such iron control required. At court, when the King and Queen were present, Fanny Burney wasn't allowed to sneeze, even with a vehement cold; if a sneeze persisted, she must oppose it with all her might, grind her teeth and let its violence break a blood vessel rather than let it out. I hold my breath but don't grind my teeth for fear of moving another part. The sneeze abates but not the wind.

Should I blame the experimental breakfast? Adding a little goat's milk yoghurt and leftover Christmas apple sauce to the usual thin layer of marmite on white bread. In truth, none of it wanted, though I'm grateful D prepares it. Was it the spoonful of apple sauce: a lump to skelter through? The tell-tale wind balloon makes its way through my guts. The fruit of that forbidden tree. Apple sauce. Just hold on.

I close my eyes.

Then it's over. All has been contained.

I go back along the corridors stepping polly wolly doodle all the day. I am tired, tired.

After time in bed, woozy but sleepless, I trundle to Father's flat to prepare for his coming. His orchids and little potted poinsettias are dead. He will be sad I've not nurtured them as he would have done. He'll show he's disappointed only by a fallen face. The plant stall in the market would close if everyone were like you, I'll say.

I should go out to buy more orchids, but have no energy: in any case, there's no McDonald's with its lovely clean toilets between here and the market. I've not actually eaten its hamburgers these 30 years, but I overflow with gratitude.

Going to Princeton once a week I used to stop at a drive-in, put my hand out and an Egg McMuffin would fall into it; then I'd drive along with a hot greasy bun in one hand, the other casually on the wheel. In Cape Coast, only good fresh palm wine and a fried plantain would get me up the steep hill to the bungalow in my clapped-out little Fiat. It could carry one person going up, not 2.

Alcohol and cars and grease, such a heady, lovely conjunction.

The sugar-cane workers from the flat coast land by Komenda piled in when I offered them a lift: chewing betel as they squashed politely into the back and little front seat. I wore a frilly pink and white check tent dress above knees that should never have been exposed. Girls weren't as pretty in the 1960s as they are now.

I haven't thought of Ghana in years but now it's almost as present as Dotheboys Hall. My first proper job, discounting underwear-selling, china-packing, plum-picking, pig-guarding, and au-pairing, was teaching in Ebenezer Rock of God School in Accra. After Cambridge, the classiest and most sophisticated joined the BBC or Foreign Office – those Cheltenham Ladies' girls I fantasised, already engaged to boys with prospects and private means – though the boys would have to wait if their girls were in the FO, since married women weren't allowed to do open diplomacy. The rest of us seemed unemployable – a touch unmarriageable too.

At the end of a long idle summer in the Shropshire village where Mother and Father now lived – Father lured into business there in part for love of A.E. Housman whom he quoted far too often – I spied a small ad for teachers in newly independent Ghana. I'd met few Africans but kept an impression of black children with multi-coloured satin bows in their hair when I stepped off the boat in Bermuda in the 1940s (my own plaits tied with drooping brown elastic). I had hopes for Ghana.

The selection was lax. The following week I was to find an African in a bowler hat at London Airport, *The Times* in his left hand. He'd give me a plane ticket to Accra. I picked up my guitar, packed a few flowery tent frocks a friend had run up for me, and left home. Mother was doubtful about the move.

'There's bound to be a British consul,' said Father.

The flight was a little shaky. I was met at the airport by a bevy of boys rather than the headmaster I'd expected – apparently he'd succumbed to palm wine and magic. They carried me to Ebenezer, then sat me down to the fieriest palm-nut soup in the world. Having experienced Ceylon curries, I passed the test but the roof of my mouth was flaming. (When, in that first night, did those pairs of dark eyes remove themselves from the crack below my window blind? I was jolted as I spied them but, when I looked at them directly, they didn't move. Just curiosity. Me too.)

Flying back to England the following year was shakier – Ghana Airlines had been abruptly Africanised and men with little training put in charge. We were supposed to land in Zurich en route for London but our pilot couldn't manage it. The plane lurched in circles, passengers hearing every word between pilot and bewildered ground control. In the end diverted to a flatter city; by which time we held tight hands with strangers. We were taken off and moved on to another quieter plane with thick tartan seats.

I'd applied to teach English Literature (not *Animal Farm* – I knew this 'reactionary' novel was banned). I was assigned French and History. The wrong history: soon informed that Nkrumah, Our Leader, had written the correct post-colonial version. 'I'll teach what I'm told,' I said to the Ministry man in suit and dark glasses who came in his Mercedes to visit my class. 'Draw a line under last week's lesson, boys.'

At least I was teaching something. Unlike, I suspect, the 2 Tanyas, who arrived from Russia a month or so after me, with hardly a word of English. We communicated mainly with smiles and nods. Extraordinary products of the Soviet system: friendly, provincial girls quite ignorant of the outside world. Lacking any sense of capitalist private property, one afternoon they simply 'found' a car. (One Tanya had driven a tractor.) They bumped it back into the compound and used it to go out in the evenings. They continued in their merry manner – sticking pictures from glamour magazines high up on their white walls and listening to sentimental Russian songs on a small gramophone with tears coursing down their cheeks – then someone from the Embassy came and removed them – possibly the car incident had been too much. I think they went back to Russia: I heard later one of them had a young child there.

When Ebenezer failed 'Osagyefo' by omitting to send Young Pioneers for his birthday parade in Black Star Square (the Headmaster deep in palm-wine haze), I was translated to another school, then a college in Cape Coast, a beautiful new place on a hill overlooking the sea. There during the coup, I hid portraits of Nkrumah (hanging in each house and classroom) in case he came back and tried to discover who'd likely spent the turbulent night scrubbing the red outline of his head off the side of the building and jettisoning his image. History has a nasty way of returning when you least expect it. Our Principal was apparently found trying to bury his big black Mercedes (the badge of all the apparatchiks) in the sand – this may have been apocryphal.

I'm grateful to Ebenezer and Bawku, Mfantsipim, Komenda and Cape Coast colleges. Without them, I'd never have had what I never dreamed of: a life *paid* to read novels. (In my world, if you liked books you became a librarian, but I wasn't quiet enough and knew next to nothing of libraries.) Criticism too I had to read, but not much written (in those days) on those loud, splendid authors who startled me out of my regurgitating life: marvellous women like Aphra Behn and Mary Wollstonecraft, the latter rejected as topic for my thesis because so very obscure. So obscure I started a newsletter to see if anyone else out there cared tuppence for this meteoric writer or her fellows, for Mary Astell, Mary Hays et al. (Many did, though not yet chaps at Yale, certainly, and not for many years anyone at Cambridge. But by then I'd had a decade of rooting down rich cultural byways, feeling the heady joy of virgin footnotes.)

Mother always thought such 'work' simply money for old rope.

When, 3 years on, I returned to England from Ghana, my parents were no longer in Housman's Shropshire and not pleased to be gone, having suffered one of the many downward slides in Father's undulating life. 'Wrong turn there,' he admitted breezily many years later.

He appreciated all his chequered life.

I look again at Father's carefully titled Book of Instructions. Underneath is a folder called 'Memories of My Dear Wife', prefaced by his sing-song poem, 'Courting in Happy Valley'. My pretty, black-haired, green-eyed mother sits on a tussock eating cherries and spitting stones into the brook, while together they watch squirrels chase up and down a hawthorn tree. (For a birthday I gave him the memoir, *Bad Blood*, by my former colleague, Lorna Sage. He recognised one of the characters: 'I stepped out with her. Lovely girl.' He didn't elaborate: nothing should interrupt the narrative of Mother's romance.)

In the tidy bedroom I see pictures of young and old mother – and of the lady who succeeded her. Nobody stayed to the end. Let's hope I do.

Going around his flat like this, it's as if he'd died. But he's not dead. He's coming home.

D picks me up and we go to fetch Father. He was supposed to have a session to see if he could boil a kettle or an egg. He can of course but no one has checked. What of the *C.difficile*, the awful runs he still has?

'Can you get out of bed unaided and dress yourself?'

'Yes.'

This is to refuse Social Services.

He's given a packet of medicines to take home.

D goes to get the car and I walk with Father. If he strolls with a lady, he takes the road side, just as he always, even in pain, gets up if someone enters the room. So weak and tired now, he insists on carrying his own bag. But I'm younger than you I say trying to take it from him, why are you insisting? He looks at me with his one eye. 'I suppose because I always have,' he says, and holds on to it.

He lives by obsolete codes of conduct. Especially courteous to the rude and indifferent. Once I watched him pick up a chocolate wrapper discarded by a young woman with bare white midriff.

'You dropped this, Madam,' he said raising his hat.

'I don't want it.'

'Neither do we.'

A little snarl but she took the wrapper.

'You'll get in trouble one day doing that,' I said.

*

When we bring him to his small sitting-room he sinks – unusually for him – into his armchair, holding his head. C has raised it on 4 rubber tubes, so it's easier to get in, and placed a special lamp nearby.

I ring the hospital. Can he have any help? His bowels are more unsteady and appalling than mine. Social Services, they tell me, gets a person out of bed and washes him. They have half an hour.

Nothing else?

No.

I see him lurch and fall about, his one eye unsteady, his jaw aching too. He's awaiting more radiotherapy on his head, for the metasta-sising skin cancer brewed so long ago in dazzling India, Bermuda, Jamaica, Uruguay, and Ceylon before sunscreen was thought of and when white men's balding pates were deemed invulnerable. Will there be time for this to travel through his jaw and squander his head? Which part of him will destroy the rest?

We're wrecks we agree. The humour's gone from our self-pity. At least you've had 30 more years, I try not to say. He interrupts my thoughts: I want to go on till August, the birthday, the Baby at one, that's all. I look doubtful, so does he.

He opens the packet of medicines from the hospital. Paracetamol and something for constipation!

Father doesn't really do self-pity, not in my way, his self-assessment being real. If his soul is ever 'sick', to echo poet William Cowper, it's for the 'wrong and outrage' of others.

'I can't stay,' I say.

3 January, Tuesday

Persuaded out to early supper last night by visiting friends. In Jamie Oliver's noisy new restaurant in the splendour of an old Cambridge bank. I reject everything my old self loved. How weird to remember and want desire and not feel it, an ontological sickness?

Nothing with chilli, no fruit, no whole grains, no nuts, no peas, just white pasta or rice. A gin and lime, just a small sip or 2. A couple of hours of good cheer interrupted by discreet trips is all I crave. But I take a premature taxi home in less than an hour.

Punished for pleasure. I spend the night in my cubicle, eyes closing between bouts of pain. I can't face any breakfast. Do taste buds atrophy in sympathy with the pelvis? Can pelvic radiation reach the mouth? Am I a whirl of rays?

If I had X-ray eyes, the room would be incandescent.

Can't even read. Ask again: why does the bottom half have such rights over the top? Body over thinking head. Why is the former fizzing with energy and the latter so enervated? A car alarm in the night not more demanding. (One thing about pain, it knocks fear right out of the frame. Not a lot of room for anxiety when the synapses are snapping so furiously.)

I stay off the Web but in the dark, too tired. Dark is a way and light is a place, boozy, wordy Dylan T again ringing in my mind – Welsh always called windbags – would Neil Kinnock have lost the general election if he'd been Scottish, not a *Welsh* windbag, a Welsh git? English gits, Scottish windbags?

Didn't Anne Robinson say What is Wales For? And didn't the EU miss it off their map?

Fat slag; thin what? Words, words. 'Never until the mankind making / Bird beast and flower . . .'

I walk the corridors as usual, absurdly on the absurd dot. The Bury people are there but no receptionist, no radios pacing by with cups of coffee. I can't be cheerful.

Worse things at sea, Father said so often. There certainly were. I have read *The Cruel Sea*. I was with the *Newcastle* and the *Highlander* and the *Glorious* . . . Stories are colliding and morphing. We wait in silence.

Someone must be called first. I want LA8 to be fresh for me. At its best.

I go in ahead of the others and heave on to the carbon fibre, then am hoisted further up. The machine will sniff round, then send forth its beams. Good, bad? If it doesn't save, it makes things worse.

I display my corpse to the great eye, motionless on my bier, my catafalque. Mourners leave, lights dim and the machine hisses, the sound like a long-drawn creak of a door shutting.

Restrain thoughts of sacrifice. Nobody sacrifices old women, just casts them out of the igloo when they're a burden. The knife's erotic: victim skin must be taut; the cheek rose and white for the mortal drama. People tend to believe the ageing *satis* in India chose their fate, not so clear with that teen-ager in Deorala, with her mass of murderous watchers. (On the English streets, youths with dreads and dogs appeal over the hunch-backed, chronic down-and-out with her urine-stained bundle.)

If I survive this, I will die Under Milk Wood, willingly, neither bad nor good. I'll have sat my time on Sir John's just hill above the fern and foxy places with the hawk on fire. Blithely squawking, green and dying, clear as a buoy's bell by Fern Hill.

After such melodrama, such visions, what could you do, Dylan T, but drink yourself to death, like the desolate boy who slits his throat? But, with moderation, avoiding gin and green beans, we can wait a little longer in your melodious lap.

Reading muddies the mind. Just as well I can't do much of it. What sort of preparation for infinity? What sort of booty in the brain? What sort of solace?

Better than the vacant mind, people often say.

Why? Is any mind vacant? I doubt it. So why be snooty?

*

It's over, I've held in the wind, with everything else. The servers return. I swivel off the couch only to remember it's raised. I nearly tumble down. The girls look a warning. A prostate enters and we nod slightly. Grey spectres passing. I huddle into clothes growing slack despite potatoes and puddings.

'Nobody wants to be in this place,' says one of the girls.

Count your blessings, name them one by one, then you will see what the Lord has done. Exactly so.

There are far worse things, far worse disabilities, far nastier fates, and to grumble when you still have – fill in the blank – is wrong. I know.

By the time I'm back in the waiting-room I'm breathless with fatigue. Once I started to write a book called *Breathless* about asthma in literature. I no longer have the heart – or lungs – for it. Cancer is bigger, all that fighting talk, that sense of rendezvousing with death.

'No one,' the games teacher used to shout at me as I wheezed up the school mountain at the back of the crocodile to F set's perpendicular playing field, 'ever died of asthma.' You just need willpower to breathe properly.

Maybe it was the drama of a well respected, solemn disease that gave me that quick stab of relief whenever I heard the cancer diagnosis: fussing is justified for a death-delivering illness which, unlike asthma, can't be mocked.

Did I think, deep down, I deserved it – not then perhaps but some time?

Or was that momentary relief just perversity, an elaborate way of coping?

I walk with D back down the almost empty corridor to the car park, visualising a comforting death. I'd move slowly, all thin and transparent or diaphanous, onwards through a misty mirror or along the sand to the blurring sea, enveloped in curling mist. Sad watchers would turn away into the clarity of the shore, morally improved by the sight, elevated as if I were Little Nell or Little Eva or Clarissa passing into A Better Place. 'I left my body on a distant shore.' Then I remember poor Mother – her skeletal, almost decomposing skull, gasping for food or drink. Was it denied? Is this what hospitals do when they need the beds – or think a body not worth keeping in breath? Or was it a brutal kindness?

Death should be slow-moving, calm, gradual, solemn. (Thinking 'consumption' of course, not cancer.) Sleep, that's the point. 'Sleep after toil, port after stormy seas,/Ease after war, death after life does greatly please,' wrote Edmund Spenser in his interminable *Faerie Queene*.

A good death was once a painful death overcome with faith; we faithless think we deserve no pain. A good death now is one that comes in secret, in sleep.

Drowning isn't painless. Radiant, self-pitying Mary Wollstonecraft jumped into the Thames, grew unconscious, then bubbled up and floated downstream. Rescued by a Society set up to lift bodies before they became corpses. If she tried suicide again, it wouldn't be through drowning, she said. Her sad elder daughter Fanny, whom I love as a daughter, took the resolve to heart when she killed herself with poison by the sea in Swansea 19 years on. 'Love' because I wrote her story and felt its sadness after such glittering promise – little 'Fannikin' enjoying a coach and scarlet waistcoat; going 'plugity plunge', eager for a special mug marked F from Stoke – yet in the back of my mind that knell for any orphaned, illegitimate child: her loving mother's shrug, 'she does not promise to be a beauty'.

After writing her life, I could never stomach praise of her vain and selfish family: cruel Shelley, arrogant half-sister Mary and spoilt, uncaring Claire. All of them watching Fanny go through Bath to avoidable death. Frankenstein's Monster – forget his gothic creation, just silly science fiction of men getting babies without women. It's what happens after that matters, the rejection, the repulse. Fanny was as outcast as Mary's Monster, but lacked his tremendous, vengeful strength. She went on loving that vicious trio when she should have blasted them to hell.

I think of von Aschenbach in his deathly deckchair on the Venice Lido, paying the price for his hidden love. A calm sea and pretty boy rising. Not bad. The Adriatic like porridge before him. (So different from that hungry sea round Wales.)

If real-life death's an exaggeration of what's happening these last weeks, it won't be calm. Dignitas, please. Can they do it long distance, at your own convenience? Can you do it online?

I'm too tired to visit Father in his flat. Others do, for he's a friendly, good natured, lovable, though talkative man. C will take him chicken soup. I ring him but as usual can't get him off the phone without an excuse. He's sad about the poinsettias and orchids. He doesn't like any living thing to die if it can be helped. He's worried about me and I about him. We coo over the Baby, then talk too much of our symptoms.

Do be quiet, I say to us both. Just keep it in.

4 January, Wednesday

Last night I had a dream – which means I slept a while. A long road stretching to somewhere. I wake up with dread. A recurrent dream of being lost and struggling to get to an unknown 'home'.

Consciously I relish an open road at the start of a journey. Dreams seem to know differently.

Dread cedes to fuzz.

On to the Web. On the trail of Stage and Grade 2 this and that, the likelihood of mortality in an operation following failed radiotherapy. I find it. But what do I need to know?

Actuaries tell it all. The lack of health insurance for travel. I seek what I won't accept. If I really knew my odds, though, I could start calculating, counting down.

It's not possible to talk sensibly to the bladder, vagina and bowels, what's left of them. They're going through too much, poor dears. The brain also is awry. A Web page lists all the possible disasters that can befall someone like me, each item says to tell your doctor.

Indeed? Would any GP, any consultant, any nurse ever pick up a phone and listen? I think not. Even if we call them Doctor over and over, genuflect, and answer to our first names like children. Why should they? Their time's limited. They can't indulge grumblers.

I haven't yet cancelled my lecture in Florida. Do planes take passengers with one hand over a mouth, the other clutching a pelvis? I ring up the airline.

'Absolutely not. Do not travel if you're unwell.'

Makes sense.

I remember Florida, 40 years back, without health insurance. In veterans' war huts moved on to the university campus from Georgia to house foreign and poor students. No medicine for asthma, no help for a baby with prickly heat in eyes and ears, weather hot as fire on the tin roofs, no air conditioning allowed – wiring would explode. Cockroaches, mosquitoes everywhere. From time to time a truck spraying clouds of DDT to fumigate our rather squalid village. Children jumping about in the spray like gleeful ghosts.

Once, as I wheezed along the road, finding no air to pull in, I and the baby fell by the wayside and were picked up, pram and all, by cops. You shouldn't be walking on a street, they said. It was a foreign habit.

They didn't take us to hospital: no insurance.

An Indian woman from Calcutta contracted meningitis and our huts were sealed off. Like a medieval plague village.

The place was bulldozed even before we left the state. But something magic there: alligators slinking along paths searching for the pastel marshmallows that rotted their teeth, anhingas hanging up their feathery wings to dry, fireflies flashing in the dark against cypresses, Spanish moss dangling from clothes-lines, and a baby splashing water in a blue plastic basin in the sunlight. Had I been able to breathe in smoke-filled seminars and dust-mited, asbestos-walled apartments, I couldn't have been more content.

I've almost stopped sleeping. So, this last night I gave up Googling cancer to chase insomnia. Looking for a link between the 2? Of course.

I read a newspaper column. I'd like to batter the author.

Insomnia, she writes, may be cured by 'someone to love'. Rot! I have good people to love. Are only 'lonely hearts' awake at 3 a.m.?

I recognise the products she promotes. Boots the Chemist adorns them with crescent moons and sleepy long-lashed eyes. Same old ingredients: passiflora, camomile, valerian, nux vomica. As if! Eat them like smarties and not a wink.

Then mogadons, temazapans, melatonin from passing Continentals, all the Zs, zopiclone and zolpidem and zalepion, delivering a few hours at most. Poppy and charms, as good as death thought John Donne. Christopher Smart believed mandragora helped gout: I've heard it's good for sleep, but chemists never stock it.

Did you know, writes this infuriating young columnist, that, if we sleep fewer than 6 hours a night – I should be so lucky, not for years – the levels of inflammatory substances in the blood can jump by 25%? The constant high levels harden arteries and damage hearts and exhaust the immune systems leaving us susceptible. To what?

Someone said insomnia comes to us at night in revenge for what we've refused to acknowledge by day.

Great: dumping on insomniacs. Like the obese.

Once, on a fellowship in Oxford, I answered a call for insomniacs. As I walked through tiled corridors in the Warneford, an inmate took my arm and hissed, 'Go away.' I don't remember much about the clinic except it didn't cure insomnia. Why should it? Insomnia's a curse – sometimes the quiet, velvet sort.

Insomniacs have more of every day when they're alive, albeit a rather gothic one.

Into Emmeline, taking my usual seat. I lean against the wooden rail at just the wrong angle to poke the back of my head. Do private patients have seats like this?

Would I be allowed into a *private* hospital in a saggy red skirt? A Groucho Marx moment.

Under the machine. The demeaning public dome of the pelvis smooth as alabaster. Shaved by fire.

For always.

I wait for the singsong to start. It doesn't come. Something's wrong. There's a pause. I'm sure the eye didn't go underneath. No one will risk coming in to turn me off. Gitche Gumee floods my mind at the end of its tether.

Just hold on to 'nice' memories, said one of the cancer books. Same old refrain. But nice memories have sauntered off.

*

I know the machine's stuck. Only half way round. I've missed some of the treatment and it's burnt only one part. Will anyone admit this? Dare I ask?

M and a young man come in at last. I hint my misgivings as I slither off so they can wipe down the top for the next victim. We patients are such scaredy-pants.

'We wouldn't send you away without finishing the process,' the young man says tartly – however degenerate the machine?

To humour me after this startling experience, they seem prone to chat. I grumble, of course. Expensive use of NHS time, but I've paid into it long enough to deserve a bit of stroking.

Why did I have to wait so long for treatment?

In France, Germany and the US, M says, it wouldn't have happened.

Always the greener grass, we all agree.

And of course there are contra-indications, caveats, etc. Who wants confused bladders and bowels? Who wants more cancer, tell me that? We might chat up here, but down below the ceaseless talk between bladder and bowels goes on and on, and the weary brain can't get a word in edgeways.

I'll never know what happened. I don't even know if the burning, the nuking, is working. The body so secretive. In Aphra Behn's long clever novel *Love-Letters*, her naughty heroine Silvia faints in the presence of her husband of convenience. When she comes round, she can't discern whether or not she's been raped. She never knows, he doesn't tell, and her body won't let on. But Richardson's villain Lovelace lacked such scruples: he raped, told, and destroyed the wonderful Clarissa.

So, there we have it: Clarissa knew, Silvia did not, although both women were unconscious. In a nutshell this is the difference between 17th- and 18th-century culture.

*

I must make a virtue of necessity. No necessity of virtue? I'm so tired, so weary of it all. Hiawatha recedes but Lovely Woman is stooping to folly over and over as I wander lonely as a cloud. And down the corridors to the car park All Things Bright and Beautiful follow me. The sky is on fire and I must go. Shut the eyes of the dead not to embarrass anyone.

'Get a grip,' I say aloud. Someone turns to look at me.

No insomnia in the grave.

Later in the day I try again to work in the office. How much longer can I hide my mashed-up brain? Am I exposing myself already? Do my colleagues snigger by the coffee machine or just wish I'd go away? They must be so bored by it. I'm tired beyond sleep. Names, never my strong point, disappear into the mist. Fearing I'd be discovered to have an IQ of 50, I never took the test. Avoiding the dementia check too: funny shapes to be remembered and words kept in sequence. No thanks. The ego is an egg and eggs break.

Cancerous men like C. Hitchens, propped up in front of their computers writing on and on, illness no way affecting their minds. But the Web says many patients feel fuzzy-minded or forgetful with disease. Not so Jane Austen, scratching away with a quill; then, when she couldn't hold a quill, with a pencil; then dictating. Some critics deplore her unfinished *Sanditon* for its silliness and degenerate style. But I love its freakish invalids and hypochondriacs who invest every mouthful of buttered toast with drama, self-medicating with wild hyperbole. Has anyone but Jane A mocked the changing hues of disease while noting them on her own body or poked fun at feebleness confined to an armchair? Not sainthood perhaps, but greatness.

Aphra too was witty — about other people's mishaps. When a fellow playwright sat in a sweating-tub for venereal disease, she rallied him with naughty comic lines. Like us pelvic irradiatees, he too was 'half-famish'd' on a diet of hard dry biscuits and 'penitential' drink, coddled every morning 'in a Cask'. His object of blame was easier than ours: 'this Female' who made him 'Spring and Fall'. Another playwright, William Wycherley, served Aphra her own medicine when he advised her, should she also be infected, to go for a sweating cure to her own plays — since they were so steamy: if 'you have need to Sweat,/ Get, (if you can) at your New Play, a Seat'.

I give up trying to read a report, let alone saying anything sensible. I go home to bed. I stay there.

Outside the day is beautiful, cold, and sunny. I notice this when getting up — over and over — I open the window for a moment on the clear air and let condensation fade. The beauty of the bare branches against the sky overwhelms me. Is this because I mightn't see it for long or because other functions have slowed and I've time to stand and stare. Or am I just slushy through weakness?

Nothing like a spot of illness to bring appreciative tears to the eyes. Ambidextrous ones, looking inside with soft pity, outside with such indulgent rapture. 'Aching joys.'

No condensation on that Welsh attic window: same temperature in as out. But the duck-feather, breath-stopping eiderdown was warm. In boarding school, sometimes ice formed along the bed-heads below an always open window. 'Cold never hurt anyone,' said Matron. I put my socks over my hands. In time, while pedalling my legs under the sheet to create warmth, I wondered about Milton's 'frozen loins' of the 'populous North', an idea I rather liked, ignorant of the difficult engendering. I never found Milton especially sexy but he was good company in a cold bed, as on a blustery moor.

5 January, Thursday

I try to avoid the World Service and Shipping Forecast by putting on Classic FM. Gustav Holst's Jupiter theme from *The Planets*: 'I vow to thee my country'. Reminded of green willow banks and rural rides, Father reminiscing of Welsh buttercup meadows and dashing brooks through soft, hot colonial evenings in places all renamed in post-colonial times.

Reminded too of a simpler age when, as a boy, he was made to take his cap off to the blind local squire and people stood up for the national anthem in little front parlours, and patriotism flourished with proper enemies of fascism and poverty. Not the same now, its implications more murky: even Father rarely speaks of England or Wales or Britain – except for rugby or cricket – just his pride and pleasure in a local place, not exactly where he's put down roots – no time for that – but where he's watched a spring struggle into being.

How lovely to sit and stare at the Great Ouse with a small flask of coffee, its cork wrapped in greaseproof paper; how joyful to see the little nursery-school children shrieking and playing ball in the park, bright clothes among the flower beds (he'd yearned for the large family Mother could never have, but got over it). 'How lucky I am,' he says.

Neither of us has flat lands in our bones, each feels that flutter of joy as England rises towards Welsh hills, but he also knows that irises are more delicate over here in these monotonous fens, the walks gentler for old old legs.

To be moved is to be ill, the healthy stand firm. Pathos is pathetic, needy. Come now, I tell myself. I leave Classic FM, happy they don't play 'The Ash Grove' to stir maudlin Welsh memories.

Soon I'm sitting on my hospital seat. No Bury couple, no cheer. I manage a few pages of *White Fang*, virile bodies and Call of the Wild. I read even more slowly than I used to, winding down like Hal in *2001* or those demented painters who paint less and less detail and slither into abstract lines. Fire flickering into grey ash. And so on. Oh 'those blue remembered hills'. How Father loved Housman – but he's stopped quoting him, not even greeting a white flower with 'wearing white for Eastertide'.

LA8 is being cleaned or serviced, or just comforted. I'm on LA5. It sticks ¾ way through. I'm suspicious again. Why is it obstinate? Afterwards the young radio man asks me about symptoms. I dislike telling a man about sticky discharge. From where exactly? Thin or thick? Well, I mumble.

I have a gurgling drain in the middle of me – no organs but a bag of floating guts. I can hear bubbling. *Hob y deri dando*. What does it mean? The pig under something? *Ar hyd y nos* goes round and round without sleep. *Calon onest* and *calon lan*.

'I feel tired,' I say.

'That's very common,' M replies, 'very common.'

6 January, Friday

In the early morning hours I listen to a tape of *The Waste Land*, drifting in and out of dozing, out enough to renew affection for a poem I used not to like. Now, among seductive words, I catch Eliot's classy contempt for uncouth accents. Mimic the buggers. A man buys his wife Lil a new set of teeth. The lower orders are *so* absurd. But that man survived the Somme. And you TSE?

The waiting-room is filled with new, loud-voiced men. One said that yesterday he drove for 50 minutes all the way here down the A14 from Bedford. He was turned away because he was full of gas. Imagine the fart when he got back into the car – or perhaps in the waiting-room before he withdrew.

I take the seat on the end, farthest from him. He'd better not be on my machine before me.

Can you believe it? LA8 is again ill-prepared – or just disobliging. I go to LA7 for the first time. It can't be right, it's a gentler, less intense machine. I worry I'm being short-changed. The girls are sympathetic but I'm glum. Full fathom five, I say to myself. Of his bones are coral made. I get through the session holding tight to every orifice. Milton's Mother Sin had trouble keeping things in: every hour she bore something nasty, then the nasties returned to howl and gnaw her bowels. *Paradise Lost* in female mode.

I go for the weekly review; I grow glummer. No one will tell me what I want to hear: you will be well. No one says I'm incorrect to moan, 'I should have been treated in June or July not December and January.' Please don't agree with me. Please say, 'They know best.'

I so want to believe in Authority, but it's a struggle. Will they write 'insubordinate' in my hospital file if I say the wrong thing?

At home I force myself to want a boiled egg despite the last catastrophe. More glum than ever. The egg smells of rationing's sulphurous dried egg. Would it all have been different if I'd eaten a macrobiotic diet, been a vegan, fasted every third day?

My first shell egg was on that first day in the First-Class dining room of Cunard's *Queen Mary*, a voyage which haunted Mother. Nothing else in a longish life quite reached that moment of peripeteia. 'Don't say you haven't seen an egg before,' she whispered across the posh silver and linen breakfast table to my 6-year-old cocky but bewildered self.

From that to this. I can't face it. But as Donne said in a better context: 'I can.'

*

'No worst, there is none,' some other chap said. But of course there always is.

I try to go into work for a few hours but feel grey and washed out, aware of my slip-slopping interior covered only by layers of cotton cloth. A gracious colleague offers coffee and biscuits. I eat a dry shortbread with water.

Prison fare. Not *modern* prisons. Luxury hotels, grumbles Father. In the war . . .

I'm beyond prison or wartime camps. I hope none of my colleagues has X-ray eyes.

I'd like a bath, but the booklet says not to use hot water and who wants a tepid tub? Bubbles not allowed either. Tepid water without drapery of bubbles. Too sad. Yet, those candle-lit baths were always better as spectacle than experience.

I try to be grateful I've reached old age, but soon give up. Sodden Dylan never reached it, can know nothing of it. No more did Keats. Shakespeare was 52, Saint Jane 41 composing funny verses on St Swithin just days before death – family thought them unseemly but we Janeites love them, believing she saw *herself* as immortal, not the rainy saint. Shelley a mere 29 in a boat with holes, having just asked, 'Then, what is Life?' – better to have asked, who put the holes there? Perhaps he knew. Byron 36, Mary Wollstonecraft 38.

All exited sharpish. Never portrayed the old from inside, just vampires sucking the young: monstrous, bestial. Or simply in the way. The toothless crone, Mr F's aunt in *Little Dorrit*, Miss Havisham, the 'loathly lady' of medieval art with her pointy nose touching her chin, the Wicked Witch.

No wonder gerontophobia exists – gerontogynophobia.

Do not let me hear of the wisdom of old men.

Nor women neither.

This is no country for old men. Much less for old women.

Ageism's the last allowable prejudice.

9 January, Monday

Before the Shipping Forecast I lie in bed – in between visits – and try to think positively, as we are told – *ad nauseam* – to do. I make an effort to conjure up a sunny National Trust property, but along comes the organic lavatory. I had to use it ahead of a woman with razored short grey hair and warm, innocent face.

I'm *so* sorry.

But what else to do? In India, in error I got on to a video bus for a 7-hour journey, the only woman, the only European, and wearing tight trousers. I learnt then that, however bad the situation, however numerous the spectators, if you face the other way, you'll get through it.

I try positive once more, using the National Trust. Attempting to visualise heritage twigs and white barks in the nearby park. Foiled again: I call up the bad-food cafeteria by the cars, awash with babies and crumbs. Rather lovely sight, actually.

It's well to have as many holds upon happiness as possible, Jane A said. Good to dwell on gladness. But no denying it's an effort.

Must have dozed then for I had an odd dream or vision of a young woman with tell-tale tattoos round the pelvis. I accosted her and grew emotional with friendliness. Then I saw the tattoos were a necklace of flowers and hearts, like barbed wire. Bit enigmatic, unassimilable.

*

As I trail back from the cubicle to bed I realise there's no going to Florida. No insurance and 10 hours on a plane. What if they closed the toilets in turbulence? What if? Nightmare. I read again in the booklet that one in 2 women will have bowel problems. They put 50% in brackets – for the fuzzy minded. I've been in the 10%, the 1 in 5,000, etc.: for sure I'll be in this half.

I look up weather in central Florida. It's 25°F and sunny. 50% bowel problems versus, shall we say, 90% sun. To be in the sun with bowel problems, not good.

And no NHS.

With all your faults, I can't leave you. My place is in Hospital-land.

I listen to the winds blowing over North Utsira and Rockall. Fair: moderate to poor.

Years ago, taking a new job in a men's college. I could find no female lavatories. I went past the smelly urinals. Should women not have drunk at dinner or have had iron bladders fitted? Apparently on Ladies' Nights when 'wives' came in, other arrangements were made.

Asked to stop a campaign bus, Margaret Thatcher is reported to have said, 'A lady needs to go only once in a day.' Iron pelvis on an Iron Lady.

Mr Cameron negotiated with the EU on a full bladder: it concentrates the mind. Did he jiggle? Did they suspect?

On with the red skirt, long socks, and blue cotton knickers, out into the dark. Through the car park and down the corridors. The Christmas decorations a memory. Now begins the mirthless part of winter. The Filipino cleaning lady huddles over her trolley staring at a holiday magazine of blue skies and million-room ziggurats on the Costas.

*

D and I arrive early at Emmeline to find LA8 in good form. No waiting. I heave on to the pyre.

The machine is a little late on one stage, but the girls will assure me there's been no hitch. Around go the square eye with its wiry eyebrows and the stealthy satellite box, making the usual hiss and wheeze.

I think of Dr Johnson with his tics and jerks and sudden lunges. How would he have faced this treatment? No one more admirable in mind, but his body would never have stayed still.

Everyone I meet and mention – I'm addicted – the Third Cancer diagnosis, tells me 'to live in the present'. Dr Johnson says that those who live in the present sit 'in the gloom of perpetual vacancy'.

I come out of the radioactive room carrying my knickers and see D sitting in a different place. He was disturbed into moving by raucous prostates and their farting stories, he whispers too loudly. Like students in Glasgow boasting they were legless, were wanked off, then passed out: great evening. As we leave I hear one man say he had so much gas in him that . . .

On the Web I look up books on death and how to deal with it. Low prices on Death and Dying, says Amazon. I go to the Library to find copies I don't have to pay for. I can't abolish thrift – even now when, surely, I could let it go. I want to be prepared – though know, from experience, I'll be taken by surprise.

People repeatedly say, Life isn't a rehearsal. Yet it's quite long; so you can try out different things. Death definitely isn't.

Some good last words ready? Friend S said her uncle, dying in hospital, observed the white-coated doctor and remarked, 'Ah the wine waiter.' You must have had a special life to rise to that.

I search out items on the Library computer. Happily the great catalogues with little stickers for titles, many handwritten in spidery script, are superseded; I'd be too weak to heave them down and up.

I begin checking. There are reams. Death Studies is a growing field. I get no further than *Preparing for Death* and Kübler-Ross on death and dying before the gurgling slackness warns me to go home without even tasting half a plain scone in the cafeteria.

In Xanadu did Kübler Ross.

I find and check out 2 books.

By the rotating door I encounter a friend who tells me her father died of lung cancer at 55. The consultant insisted his patient exercise when there was no hope. Surely cosseting and kindness would have been better, my friend thought. When she confronted him, the consultant said it was his business to be positive.

Shakespeare's Prospero thought of death a third of the time, after he'd married off daughter Miranda, finished his 'revels', and taken his revenge. Why didn't he think of it *all* the time?

At home lying in bed I study *Preparing for Death*. Apparently when the self leaves the body, the electricity within stops. There's no biochemical reception. The mind simply evaporates. This doesn't mean that consciousness of the self fails: the desires, goals, objectives and direction of the self continue to exist; they move with the self as an 'aroma' lives with a person's body.

What?

I turn to Kübler-Ross, who interviewed the dying – but not the dead, or maybe she did: she believed in spiritualism. There are 5 stages of dying. Denial, anger, bargaining, depression, acceptance. According to Wilhelm Reich, Freud got cancer when he yielded to resignation and just shrank. Best stay in the early phase.

*

I've done them all already. Maybe not acceptance. What's to accept? Not Being? You can only know afterwards.

More satisfying to think of other people's death: the brisk manner in which Saint Jane dealt with the needs of her flimsy plots, killing off characters unloved like fat Mrs Musgrove's worthless son Dick, or in the way like greedy Dr Grant, clogging up the Mansfield rectory needed for superior, younger folk. Mrs Churchill from *Emma*, who, hated for 25 years, was, when dead, 'spoken of with compassionate allowances'. She'd been judged selfish with her imaginary illnesses, but 'the event acquitted her'.

'Told you so,' she might have said, if Jane A had had the courage to follow her character's 'aroma'.

10 January, Tuesday

I have an earlier session today since someone wanted *my* slot. I negotiated down to 7.45 from 7.40, so I assume they'll like me to arrive promptly. Not sleeping, so why not go?

At 7.35 I pass by the Blood room – someone once came out remarking 'the blood's flowing easily today' – they truly did – then the bicycle poem and a couple of prostates reading tabloids. No one at the reception desk. I walk over towards LA8 to check if it's ready. An attendant snaps at me. I shouldn't be there; they're preparing the machines. I sit down, sad and tired. I'm not a natural for rules but in Hospital-land I wanted to affect a detached compliance with everything. I wanted to be politely 'subordinate'.

I don't get under LA8 till near 8 o'clock. There's music on, raw beat and synthesised wail. The girl offers to turn it off but I don't insist, chastened by the rebuke. Also, I fear to appear snooty.

Above the sound I listen to the machine's old refrain – the 3 casual slouching notes, down, up and medium, then the shrug into the relaxing, dismissing wheeze.

The notes are the 3 notes of the second phrase of 'The Yellow Rose of Texas', which sometimes I played with frozen fingers on very early black mornings in Wales instead of 'Pieces by the Masters suitable for Grade 3'. Until a brown-clad teacher raged like a grizzly bear at the door of the little room: She Could Not Stand It A Moment Longer. Not *Paradise Lost* this time but a 100 lines: 'I must not murder music.'

'I'm a martyr to music,' said Mrs Organ Morgan. Up every night till midnight playing the organ and hardly a wink of sleep. Ocky Milkman kept his wife in the cupboard with the empties.

I lie under Milk Wood.

Closing eyes against the red light. Think of *nice* memories, forget the dirty nurse of experience. So here I go again. Give up on the National Trust. Try journeys. Journeys are good – though they don't always deposit you in good places.

Many in a long life – though nothing to scurrying through the Battle of the Atlantic, freezing on Scapa Flow and scampering out of Singapore. Not that Father ever put it like this. I know, I know. But I went down the St Lawrence towards Liverpool with you breaking the ice, to Bermuda on the *Queen of Bermuda*, to Jamaica on the *Ruahine* (I think) and across the Atlantic on the *Empress of France* in a gale, though this was tame, almost tourism, to what you felt and saw. I know.

Still, you were not there when I went along the African coast through Sierra Leone and Gambia with all my belongings but no money – Ghana invented a new currency unwanted by anyone outside its borders – nor through Upper Volta and Mali to Timbuctoo in the dry season, exhilarated by all that rhythmic, red-rutted distance.

These journeys don't swim in my mind like the great one, the splendid one that jolted and smashed and anchored me into Dotheboys Hall, the one with Mother when I was 11.

Down first to Colombo along a straight road smelling of buffalo to find only one other passenger, a woman with a black moustache who was improbably named Carmen. She seemed old, perhaps about 40 like Mother. Portly with very blackened eyes. Mother was thin, pretty and spiky, and much admired, her looks being in unison with the times. She wore high black or red heels or very whitened sandals depending on season, and flared light-coloured skirts from pinch-banded waists. (She was dutiful towards me – mothers weren't demonstrative in those days.) Otherwise, only men on this shabby fleet-auxiliary vessel – appropriately neither Queen nor Empress, but just a Ranger. Chinese crew, British officers, one fair and bronzed called Gerry.

'He looks like Leslie Howard,' said Mother when she spied him.

I didn't know Leslie Howard. He wasn't in *Bambi*, the only film I remembered.

We sailed off, leaving behind my Classic Comics, *Our Island Story*, the small shelf of pre-war and wartime bestsellers I'd gorged on, the jack-al-dog, the stripy chipmunk, the black-and-white-checked tortoise called Toby, and Pat, an affectionate friend from over the harbour with whom I sometimes sat on our ramshackle jetty watching coloured fish jerk back and forth. In my suitcase an old winter coat with velvet elbow patches from years before, too short and too small, but I must have a uniform when we arrived, so it didn't matter. I was travelling to an Enid Blyton boarding school where George and Anne from the Famous Five would be my jolly chums in stained-glass halls and I'd be the heroine. (Fortunately, Mother knew nothing of the classy superiority of Angela Brazil over Enid Blyton, or I'd have had even wilder expectations.)

*

We motored along pleasantly through the Indian Ocean in white heat. Mother would pat her forehead with a handkerchief underneath her white-framed dark glasses and sometimes I'd lift up my gingham check blouse to wipe the sweat off under my beginning breasts. I was already chubby.

In the early weeks I sat on the very bow of the boat, legs dangling over the edge, gazing at flying fish on the blue-green sea. (*Titanic* spoilt the image, but I have the original.) The heat grew and grew.

The captain put a hosepipe round one of the decks, pierced holes, and forced water out. Blissful to be wet with tingling moments of cool.

Then it stopped. We were too near the Somali coast. Savages there, the captain said: they'll think we're making rain and pursue us. So we sweated again.

Carmen grumbled about everything.

Up the oily sea past the treacherous parts. It was Mother's birthday and the Chinese cook, who used to smile at me when I heaved myself up to balance on some piece of salty equipment, hoping for a little admiration, made her a cake with candles, and all the officers but not Carmen, who was either sulking or sick, came out and clapped and sang Happy Birthday. Gerry sang loudly.

I was told to take a picture of the cook and the cake with my Box Brownie camera, which I did.

Then we slid panting into Aden, all rock and nothing. We changed crew and the quiet, polite Chinese trooped off. On came scruffy dark Maltese, with cloth bundles and sagging leather cases. The captain said the women should no longer go all over the ship, and the Child should avoid the crew's quarters.

We travelled on up the Red Sea to Egypt. I leant on the rail as we got into the Bitter Lake. Dark robed men came close by in rowing boats, shaking fists and yelling 'Filthy British'. I waved and Mother pulled me away by my plaits. I watched out of the cabin porthole as more and more arrived. Soon we were surrounded by little boats of shouting, gesticulating men, some had sticks, some rifles. Among them a few held up rugs and coloured blankets to sell.

'Stay in the cabin,' commanded Mother but she went out to see.

We were shunted into a backwater. Other ships from more favoured nations sailed past through the Suez Canal. Ours wasn't pretty and it wasn't the *Queen Mary* or the *Empress of France* but I thought this treatment rude. It was hot and stuffy in the cabin, I longed to jump into the water and swim like I used to do from the jetty right round Plantain Point to where I could squirm into the tangled mangroves and be quite secret with the water monitors who slept at night under our house.

At last, after sweltering weeks in the Lake with nothing but tinned food, a final volley of obscenities and a firing of guns from the bobbing boats, we straggled out into the Mediterranean. Everyone was tired and disgruntled; we would rest in Malta. We entered the harbour, full already of British ships. I stayed mainly at the front or back. I wanted to see everything.

In the evening I was 'aft' with Gerry's cockney friend, who was holding the ensign as a great piping went up throughout the harbour. I used to chat with him but rarely understood what he said. The flag had to be taken down in a sort of goodnight ritual with other boats. A messenger came to tell him the captain wanted him. He handed the rope to me and said – I think – 'Take it down slowly when the other ensigns go down. You can't go wrong.' Off he went.

The rope was like a leash on a scampering dog, but wet and salty. Actually, 2 ropes. I had no idea which took the flag up, which down. The piping grew louder and circled round me. I could see other flags descending sedately towards the water. I tried to let one rope go slacker but it pulled too hard. No one was by to help except a Maltese crewman who simply grinned. He had hardly any teeth. The piping was coming to its end, and the other flags were nearly down while mine still flapped against the twilit sky.

I let go one of the ropes, which slid fast through my hand taking off some skin. It fell like a rag into the sea. I clutched the other rope hoping to haul the flag up but it was too sodden and heavy.

The cockney sailor came back, spluttered something to my ear, and grabbed the ropes. He might have said and done a lot worse had not Mother and Carmen come on deck just then.

That night the admiral was invited to dinner onboard to hear of our trials in Egypt. My flopping flag made a funny story. They laughed and drank a lot. I went to bed early.

Next morning Gerry, Mother and I to Valetta. What happened to Carmen? She and Mother weren't on good terms. She said, and I suppose I was meant to hear it, that I was not a polite child and was 'ungainly', an adjective much used about me in those days. So I didn't care where she was.

The dry land was lovely, the cobbles moved under our feet for we'd been so very long floating about; there were houses and little shops and an air of festivity. Gerry bought me an ice cream and pressed some money in my hand – 5 shillings I think though that sounds a lot, perhaps it was a shilling. 'Just go away for a while,' he said. I stood there while Mother studied some twisted Greek jewellery in a stall. Gerry stared at me. 'Go away,' he said again. 'We'll find you.'

I was a bit perplexed but I did go. Or *they* went. I wandered round till it was almost dark. I never spent the money: I thought I might need it to get to Wales if they didn't come back. They were quite cheerful when they did and Gerry bought me another ice cream.

Things got worse. The Maltese departed with their bags and neck chains. On came a British crew. Like pirates from *Treasure Island*.

One even had an eye patch. 'The women and the Child' were told to stay close to the cabin and to lock doors every night.

We stopped at Gibraltar and Mother made me take another snap with my Box Brownie. It didn't turn out as well as the Chinese cake.

Then we went north. I was quite excited, thinking of tuck boxes and pillow fights in that Enid Blyton boarding school.

It grew colder. We no longer sweated like pigs and needed fake rain. I didn't like being locked in the cabin but Mother said I had to be and that was that.

I began at last to read *Pride and Prejudice*, which was on board in a little library of tattered leftover books, mainly on deep-sea fishing and tropical medicine. I hadn't particularly liked it in Classic Comics and couldn't get through it. I didn't care about 5 girls trying to get married instead of going on adventures or being turbulent. Instead, I read Mother's *Precious Bane* (Milton reaching out again, though I didn't know it: the soil of hell grows riches, he wrote, the 'precious bane'.) It was almost as good as *The Sun is My Undoing*, my favourite book until knocked sideways a few years later by *The Brothers Karamazov* with its boisterous crazy men and batty women. I think I'd have appreciated *Frankenstein*, if it'd been on offer, but it wasn't yet a classic – thank feminism for that – and I hadn't seen its horrid progeny of films – indeed any horror film, unless one counts *Bambi*.

One dismal drizzly morning Gerry banged at our cabin door. 'Come out, we're aground.' We felt a bit lopsided but this wasn't unusual for such a decrepit boat. Mother laughed and said, 'That's a fine way to gain entry.' He laughed too but said it was serious.

A bit more banter which I sniffed at, then Mother put on her black and pink velvet wrap and we unlocked the door. It was just coming up to morning and the ship was certainly at an odder angle than usual. Difficult to stand up. Gerry had gone, summoned somewhere, and we were all beached on a sandbank. The Goodwin Sands apparently.

Carmen came out of her cabin, snorted, and said the whole thing was a series of errors and bungles from start to finish and, for her part, she had no trust whatsoever in this captain or his officers.

Gerry returned and pushed her aside. 'We may have to abandon ship for a time,' he said. This sounded wonderful, except that by now the water wasn't lovely and sparkling as in *Treasure Island*.

We didn't jump off. We waited, all tipped up, and at next high tide the boat shuffled back on to the sea.

It sailed up the cold coast of England to Immingham by Hull. The water was grey and greasy and people looked poor, drab and pinched. Our clothes were too thin and I couldn't get into the coat we'd brought along. Carmen scoffed and went off to London.

Mother was cross. Fed up, she said, but not why. She cheered up as we chugged in the train to Wales. And why not? She knew she'd go away soon. She was booked to leave on a better ship, a proper Cunard passenger one to India with a captain's table and snooker room. I wasn't so lucky. I wanted her to stay dreadfully. Or take me back. She was sad for me too.

16 in the dormitory, 2 rows of 8. I discovered the girls in the next beds spoke Welsh. The schoolmaster in Ceylon was mostly drunk, picked up from time to time in the monsoon drain near Plantain Point, but . . . to walk home alone through the palm and paw paw trees past the screeching monkeys on ledges on the dagoba as if they'd booked rooms in a simian hostel and didn't like them, to arrive to a pet chipmunk and a check tortoise; then to angle with a hook made from a pin for sergeant majors and multi-coloured parrot fish with crimson bellies on the end of the broken jetty, with only a jackal-dog for company. Lucifer tumbling from heaven was nothing to this change.

*

Does it sound much now? Young and retired alike go to Mauritius for a weekend, Antarctica for an anniversary. But this was a journey when the world and I were young. Places startled, not echoed: animals and people were wild, not acting wild. Nothing was packaged. Father would say he fished bodies out of the cold sea round ships that went down from the Atlantic to the Pacific when the world was still younger and far more uncomfortable. And he'd be right. Yes, but he hadn't been in the Garden of Eden at 11. Tom Paine said the serpent who entered Eden was Government; it intruded when the innocents had been perfectly happy. Read British Boarding School for Government.

A sudden swirl in the pelvic area ends my effort at positive memory – fear, like Zen's red-hot coal stuck in your rear instead of the thorax. I hold my breath, breathe and hold my breath again. The green light shimmers and the girls enter. I get down and urgency retreats.

The nurse who'd been sharp with me by the machines remarks that I look tired. I shouldn't work so hard. Did I say I was 'working'?

'Most people stop work when they go through this,' she says.

'Do you read in the night?' asks a friend. I don't (nor do I go south in the summer – no one lives in the glittering Waste Land). I do nothing but wonder and wander around aimlessly in the house, happy that there's a toilet on each floor. She suggests a holiday.

Leave the machines? Does she joke?

For lunch I risk a quarter of a ripe pear. What's left when skin and putrescent part are shaved off.

It's a bad idea.

I realise that, if I sit in my cubicle with my feet on unsold copies of *Death and the Maidens,* I can double over when spasms pass through. By the end of the afternoon I'm so tired I don't know if I'm dreaming or conscious. I hold my skull as it empties itself.

Durkheim said old women don't commit suicide because they don't have enough inner life to despair: a cat makes them happy.

Gertrude Stein's dog was better dressed than she was.

11 January, Wednesday

On the early-morning Web I come across a gem: 'after surgery, chemotherapy or radiation therapy – or simply as a result of disease in the abdomen or pelvis – an abnormal tubelike connection called a fistula can form between internal organs such as the bladder and the vagina.' Imagine! The wounded pair making merry union. Have they no care for the issue?

Back in Emmeline, LA8 is having its weekly review. I'm assigned to LA1. Music thudding. As I get on the couch and pull down my knickers I feel the strange nakedness. I'm turning into my own marble monument.

I'm prodded as usual into the most uncomfortable position, so that the coccyx digs into resisting fibre. Too timid to protest.

And embarrassed, knowing there are Stage IV people out there who'd be glad of a little bone pain.

LA1 seems to stick on the right side. Perhaps this is where most flesh is and its rays have more trouble penetrating. The machine sings its little tune. I close my eyes against the bright light, waiting for LA1 to come round to darken and deepen it.

The arch druid and whacky Welsh nationalist, William Price, burned his dead babies on a pyre, believing it an old Celtic tradition. Not to the taste of the authorities, who arrested him. He fought back.

Through his efforts cremation became a timely option in Britain: a good one given the space graves demand and our failure to recycle ourselves.

Diogenes suggested his body should become dog meat.

I feel myself slowly moving in my coffin through the curtains to the bonfire. I know there's no fire right away: they must wait and have a proper conflagration of all the corpses later. (As with those piles of slaughtered cows down leafy lanes. They can't take all that trouble for just one. We're not Hindus.) Now there are other bodies round me, and I fit quietly among them, so it will soon be time.

I open my eyes before this goes further.

Something is wrong again. The machine is stopping on its last quarter. It buzzes a little, then falls silent, buzzes once more, but it isn't adding up to the usual amount. Again, I'm suspicious.

At the end, when I tentatively ask, the radio-girls tell me I've had all the treatment. What can they say? Not 'You are losing power' or 'Sorry we nuked you.' Soon I should shine in the dark.

The Bury man and I share a predicament. They suggested Dioralyte to him. I mention the matter now, holding my knickers in place as I do so: the elastic is slack for they've gone up and down so often – or there's less of me than there was. No, say the girls, it won't do for you. You have radiation-induced problems and it would make things worse. You have proctitis, not colitis. So that's OK then?

I'm so thirsty, my mouth's a quarry, every swallow a dynamite assault. I'm reduced to Ribena, which I seek in the hospital shop on the way out. Virtuously I pick up a sugar-free carton. Encountering this elderly bag lady, the young man behind the counter warns, 'You won't like it – I should get the sugar one, love.' He's right. I replace and pay. It tastes vile, what would it have been without sugar?

I pass Costa and look for something to eat with this sticky liquid.

Not allowed nuts or fruit – but how many blueberries went into that muffin? – yet I must be careful, be kind to my tummy, as the radio-girls put it. I give it a chocolate muffin. It's stale and inedible. I take a bite and leave it. Absentmindedly, D finishes it off.

I visit the toilet cubicles on the way to the car – they have 2 main doors: in one way, out the other. Good thing, makes one feel progress.

By way of McDonald's to visit Father. Alone in his flat with his hospital-donated *C.diff.* I take him a kilo of porridge oats which he seems to think will help. He's afraid to go out.

There's been no follow-up at all from the hospital or any advice on how to cope with his problem. But, though I've been told to avoid them, he believes in oats.

Diarrhoea stops at the Scottish border? (Certainly it must further north. That old Aberdeen habit of students depositing home-made porridge in porridge drawers to last out a winter.)

I tell Father he should move on to cornflakes, no fibre there, and no food at all, but he *must* learn for himself. He's fussing about his sore teeth and pointing to them, clutching his stomach.

We're such *mementi mori*, he and I. Both of us with mouths sand-papered dry, horrid to see and feel.

Being resourceful, Father's found a spray that he's asked one of his many young friends to bring in. But I keep gulping water. This leads to problems. Am so tired it's hard to go home.

'You might pass by the park,' he says. 'There could be something coming up.'

I hug Father and feel him scrawny where he was once so firm, so definite. With all this emphasis on myself, have I failed to see his fast diminishing?

I avoid the park and go back via McDonald's, my House of Ease. I notice a mother with two small wriggling children sharing out a carton of chips. A vain young girl sways and scoops her hair from side to side. It's unbearably moving.

Out for a short early dinner with friend H from the hospital. I have a morbid interest in her work. 'You're not dying yet,' she says.

'Yet'? I jump on the word.

By way of conversation she gives examples of where she'd at first misread scans. It's common of course, common to be human. With hindsight, she says. Hindsight, like back legs with sharp eyes.

I have a small glass of red wine, small steak and small baked potato. I don't eat much of the meat, drink only a mouthful or so of the wine.

At home I go straight to bed. Just as the night time Shipping Forecast moves to the Inshore Waters I pay for the treat. I sit in my cupboard. 'Shitting Forecast,' Tucker called it in *The Loop*.

The radiator's gone cold for the night. I intend to be back in bed in time to switch the radio off as the drums begin to roll for the national anthem. I miss the moment, concentrating on other things. By the time I'm back in bed the World Service is well under way, chatting about primaries and salmons or Salmonds in Scotland. If anything should get me to sleep this should, but no. My eyes too tired to read Kübler-Ross.

12 January, Thursday

The news says that half a million children are unhappy between the ages of 8 and 16, and the government will do something about it. Legislating for happiness? Are children *supposed* to be happy? Is it a duty? A right? Must parents ensure it? Who's to blame for this rash of childish ennui?

It's America's fault with its 'purfuit of happiness' enshrined in law. My happiness is now a replenished water jug and solitude.

*

I put on my cancer uniform. When this is over, I'll cut up the red skirt for dusters.

As D and I leave the house in the dark, we hear birds singing as if spring had come. There's no more light. The world's giving out mixed messages. But, just possibly, the dark is mellowing.

I'm in hospital on time. D goes off to find a coffee. I wait with the prostates. I read *White Fang*. If I knew how to download books into phones, I'd not have come to this, but my head is soft and flaky, incapable of new skills. The message is that the strong must prey on the weak, the weak must defer to the strong. I am here with my faltering body.

'2 more days to go,' says the girl but she's wrong. '2 weeks,' says the radio man. Then it will be over. Though it never is, is it? The 'tax of quick alarm' is levied on all who have had one diagnosis.

I lie down, tailbone aching against the hard surface, the marble dome of me blurred by myopia. Language isn't catching what I feel in mind or body. Nor would it be seemly to try.

But we in Hospital-land are clinically unseemly. Take diarrhoea, that embarrassing, excremental horror, so impossible and improper to discuss. Yet a hospital form asks – po-faced – whether, for you, it comes fluid, lumpy, watery, greasy, or frothy. Best not consider its almost audible progress from one vault to another, the insecurity it causes the fart. The brain would be better off ignorant, but less wise.

Best also control the mad impulse that insists on expressing it. Father would be saddened at such unladylike revelation – or rather he'd say – doubtfully – 'Do what you think best.' As if I ever know.

It's no good. Illness bores can't stop themselves, they have to tell. They go on far longer than the Ancient Mariner and lack his glitter.

D says (humorously but . . .) a Swiftian shamelessness has come over me in these radiation weeks. More discretion might be good.

Too right. I may come to resemble Chloe from Swift's poem,

'Strephon and Chloe'. Stripped of romantic decorum on their wedding night by eating beans and drinking 12 cups of tea, the lovers reject the decent drapery of their former elegant pastoral existence; they stink along together into comfortable, unseemly marital life.

Not quite equal of course. What may be comic in men isn't in women: all authorities direct, says Swift, the most scatological of authors, that Women must be Decent. Chloe affronts propriety more than Strephon.

Virginia Woolf is with me, knowing well the 'childish outspokenness in illness' against 'the cautious respectability of health'. How little EngLit does for the sick: 'let a sufferer try to describe a pain in his head to a doctor and language at once runs down.' Truer still of bowels and bladder. 'The experience cannot be imparted.'

The fridge is singing the same 3 notes as the machine. Can this be? I lean my cheek against its cold murmur.

13 January, Friday

I lie awake in the dark between visits to . . . Hardly worth the wearying effort of trying to sleep.

Next week begins the final treatment which may have nastier effects, M says. Nastier?

'Nasty' used to mean only foul or dirty.

We set off a bit later than usual this morning. D has been up working for an hour or so already. He sneezes all the way. Why? I ask. 'Wagner and King Ludwig,' he says – when he opened their letters, the mould dust and mustiness overpowered him.

*

The day goes as it should. LA8 behaves, M attends with one girl I haven't seen before — a Tasha? Rather pretty with high brooding cheekbones, different from the moon faces of the other girls. Grushenka, beloved by feuding Karamazovs.

On the couch with the square eye coming towards me, I try to dispel dread by recalling some of the better people who've lived with me over my working years, when, for the first time, women were wanted — first as decorative sop to fashion, but then — well, you know how encroaching women can be! Mary and Fanny Wollstonecraft, and plucky Mary Hays. 3 suicide attempts, one successful, acres of unrequited love, losses, and yearnings for a world not in being and which, perhaps, wouldn't much have helped if it had been; deaths everywhere.

Idealistic, unfortunate women who caught the pulse of female feeling, spoke with a new voice.

Feminism can do much, my lord, but it cannot make bad luck good.

As for me: it rescued my life, intellectually speaking, then fractured it. (The last generation shaped before it took hold; for us it might always have been paper-thin, the old grooves too deep.) It startled me from earlier clichés of wifely, post-war femininity, but perhaps thwarted deeper thinking of consciousness, of humanity.

No tragedy there. Most thinking's ultimately in quotation marks, left on or erased.

I push out my earnest women and conjure up someone better for time-travelling: cheery, bibulous, talkative Aphra, the cleverest of them, as clever as Jane A herself and less amenable to bric-a-brac and cream teas in Bath and Philadelphia.

Once I dreamt of sailing down the Surinam river to find her. Doubtful now. Probably disappointing: there'd have been no handsome royal slave in the swamps, no tigers where they'd never been.

A brilliant playwright and hopeless spy: another agent watched her in Flanders scattering King Charles's secrets left and right, spending more money than she had – or than His Majesty proposed to send. 'Tho wrackt with various paines yet life does please/Much more than death, which all our pressures ease.' That's Aphra.

A quick review after a long wait. Too sympathetic L suggests PRADA. Not the fashion house but Pelvic Radiation Damage Association.

I go out into the air. Hope rises, for the sun is shining on frosty grass again, making it dappled in one place, twinkling in another. A low sun as of midwinter. Slight mist. A little smoggy.

With a weekend approaching I allow myself a cup of weak Costa coffee and a hot, soft, unprepossessing chocolate whirl. I want transgression. But neither coffee nor whirl tastes as it used to. I push on and achieve a few bites and sips.

I arrive home – just in time. I lean against the warm radiator. Little joys forbidden. No eating fruit buns with raspberry jam on blue china plates in a tablecloth café. If I gave up everything, would you . . . ? But I'm way past the bargaining stage of Kübler-Ross.

16 January, Monday

In gloomy mood. I read the Pelvic Radiotherapy booklet from the hospital. You must always cover up the part; smear it in lotion, we suggest E 45; never let the sun's rays go near what has already been irradiated almost to death.

Poor Father with his head like volcanic craters has been damaged by the sun. Too many distinguished visitors to ex colonies demanding white men stand in respectful discomfort without pith helmets, showing the locals how to act. (In fact, a newspaper noted with disgust that, for the Commonwealth Royal Tour of 1954, while welcoming natives always wore trousers, *some* British men were in shorts – including Father, whom Mother thought dapper in his starched white with long white socks.) We'd been following the Royal Party in heat and rain from Colombo to Anuradhapura, Polonnaruwa, Sigirya and Kandy for the final great elephant Perahera – not primarily for elephants, but I remember them trundling by on their huge feet with fire gleaming in high eyes – and Father might be forgiven for wilting into informality by the close.

Why did *I* have to wear white gloves since I never shook the regal hand? Better than the black Welsh stovepipe hat I wore in the rain 2 years before with children from the Council School, waving a red dragon flag at the royal car hurtling by unseeing towards the new Claerwen dam. Aunty baked special crown fairy cakes and the station spruced itself with panels and a 'royal toilet' – sadly ungraced by the royal posterior. Festivities concluded, there was much jockeying among locals to sit on it – the newsreel I noticed called us 'Welsh country folk'. Hinting too at sabotage. Long before Sons of Glyndŵr began burning holiday cottages: but there was bitterness at this flooding of Welsh valleys for the benefit of England.

The sun was Father's undoing, to adapt M. Steen's pretentious title. Previous occupants of the Ceylon house left the book behind. I devoured it before setting sail, remembering even now every detail – as clearly as I remember the gestures in Classic Comics' *Wuthering Heights* and *Jane Eyre*. Though anti-slavery, *The Sun is My Undoing* is flamboyantly racist; so, like so much of my earlier life, difficult to discuss. (A novel which, in Dorothy Parker's attributed words, is 'not to be thrown aside lightly. It should be thrown aside with great force.' But too late.) Years ago, the brilliant, pugnacious Indian scholar in America, Gayatri Chakravorty Spivak, remarked that whatever I said would never carry the weight of what *she* said, the Times being on her side – never mind class and money, race was the thing. She was right, the world moved on from my part-colonial childhood.

But I left it too soon; for me it was caught in shining amber, no required amnesia quite smashed it.

At Cambridge I read Franz Fanon's *Wretched of the Earth* and thought – retrospectively – it was improper to have attended a Bermudan school for girls of European descent – though at 7 I noted only its lavishness in contrast to the prefab over the bombsite, my first real school in Plymouth. Incorrect to have a mind stocked with horror at the Black Hole of Calcutta and relief at lifting the Siege of Lucknow: Dinna ye hear the piping Campbells?

Yet, it was difficult to judge Father and his unanalysed benevolence wherever we were. His efforts before we left Ceylon to send his Tamil workers to the Gulf to avoid a bloodbath – it came later; preventing a ship from sailing after its drunken British crew urinated on a local bartender – no excusable high jinks after too long at sea, he insisted to the irate captain, just horrid behaviour for which they must pay.

He understood the Winds of Change ending the British Empire, accepting the world turns only one way. Yet, though he showed no religiosity of remembrance, he never questioned imperial ethics of the past: jogging along with the times wherever they went.

Mother, perhaps, stayed in Marguerite Steen, so relieved when, instead of marrying a suitable Ghanaian, I turned (disastrously – one had to marry someone and soon) to a handsome white American of 'good' family with whom I shared almost nothing. (When encountered, the 'good' family proved menacingly eccentric.) 'One thing for the daughter of Sir Stafford Cripps to shock the country by marrying an African chief,' said Mother, 'quite another for you.' Cripps was a rich Labour politician – socialism and privilege always combined in Mother's mind: they went with a liking for expensive artisan mugs instead of china teacups, and habitual wine with meals.

Throughout her life she voted for the party of David Lloyd George as if he were still the boy from Llanystundwy.

On the bit of Radio 4 news I hear before we leave this morning, I learn we shouldn't eat processed meats and sausages because they cause pancreatic cancer. More reasons for cancer, the onus always on the diseased. Do they never stop? Irritated, I'm yet in tune with the national mood. We're all looking for the cause. In this report, blame falls on wicked foodstuffs, but also on *us*: something we did.

But we who sit by LA8 have been blameless, or almost. We've not sucked on cigarettes, we're not obese, we're not alcoholic, we don't over-consume sausages or salami or eat imprudently or live in demonstrable pollution. Blame elsewhere. I feel murderous towards Consultant X.

Slap hand, shut eyes whenever I plan a future. There's a hostage to fortune for sure. Lakshmi, always ready to tip your boat over when the sea's the calmest, La Belle Dame Sans Merci. Memory's safer. You can't jinx the past.

But you can vary it. Memories are stories too, shared and cut about to make new tales, never quite reliable, furring at edges. I had you under a table in a basket in Plymouth as bombs fell and demolished houses, said Mother; in the day we walked up and down the streets, come wind or rain, because the landlady hated children, especially ones that wheezed and were sick in the night.

I don't remember this, though she mentioned it often enough, always ending with our flight in a blacked-out train back to Mid-Wales where, unless manically off-course, the Luftwaffe was unlikely to drop its load – (how much did she regret her jolly life at ICI with a pack of giggling, dancing girls before pregnancy intervened? Father's retelling accommodated the time to his more heartening, valiant vision. Over 6 years apart in their young lives, fair enough for both to make the 'truth' expedient.)

Father sent home an exquisite frock for a girl-child he hadn't seen, obviously chosen by a dubious female in some faraway port, thought Mother – I called it a fairy frock and was rarely allowed to wear it. Then, when I was nearly 4, my cheery, unknown father came home and put his naval cap on my head for fun. He noted my first words to him: 'Where's Annabel?' But that's only *his* memory.

I liked the Florentine china doll, kept so carefully in its felt bag, but it was never my bedtime friend. Instead each night I hugged a real stuffed tortoise whose feet came loose from the board through too much caressing. I loved the hard spiky dead thing.

Mother and I watched the London victory parade on Pathé news because Father was marching in the front row. He kept his eyes straight ahead as the others turned theirs towards the King. I dropped my ice cream at the very moment he passed and so missed him. You don't read about the victory parade now. The wrong people marching? Poles were omitted – was anything else incorrect?

Some memories are patchily clear, kaleidoscopic. Comfortable deaf Aunty. During rationing you kept scraps for me from the elderly evacuated lodgers, although we knew they'd ask for them again next day and you'd pretend they'd been thrown away by mistake or, since they were growing senile, been already eaten. I still feel the fug in your warm kitchen below the street where we saw only shoes going by on the pavement and the rain pounding puddles. (Decades later when I visited Wales from America and you lived in just a floor of the dampening house, you'd come puffing up the hill to where Mother and Father lived – after yet another move – carrying a little basket of sweets and Mars bars for my children, entwined with plastic flowers: since you thought I disapproved with my American ways, you'd cover the offering with a layer of apples and pears, which they gleefully pushed aside.)

One day early in 1949 Mother danced down the basement stairs clutching a letter from Father, singing that we were – Father, Mother, and the Child – going to Bermuda right now to live and it would be paradise. And it was. But she had to cut up the curtains in the little back sitting-room to make evening dresses, for we were (unaccountably) travelling first class on the *Queen Mary* with diplomats, ambassadors, ministers and rich women quite out of our normal sphere. People who knew nothing of scraps from other people's plates or cut-up curtains. (The stuff a little singed where a candle had caught it one dark Christmas.)

The 'insubordination' marring reports from my boarding and posh schools must have come later, for I impressed these rich, important people with my polite manners. So that, when Easter came, they gave me – the only child in sight – eggs made of real chocolate instead of tin or cardboard. Mother was thin-lipped at my windfall till we came to New York and found we had a hotel booked but no dollars – nothing to eat beyond a breakfast of toast and coffee. I was indignant as she rationed out my Easter eggs between the 3 of us. We stood in front of the Empire State Building, unable to pay to go up. I think Mother hoped my newly discovered charm would appeal to a passer-by who'd want me to see inside. But it didn't.

We arrived in Bermuda full of chocolate – and probably constipated. 'It's fairyland,' said Mother. Chocolate forever, sun and pink sands and a big, white-roofed house with a sloping lawn, bougainvillea up the veranda, a swing from a cedar tree and a toad in a hole underneath, no more long, dark, asthmatic nights.

Why on earth didn't we stay for a life of beach parties and cedarwood dancing in balmy evenings? Maybe Father was restless, perhaps we all were, never quite believing ourselves part of the colonial elite that welcomed us. I visited Bermuda recently – to lecture on Jane Austen – why 19th-century American male writers hated her, or said they did. Still beautiful in a tourist-brochure way, though more built-over. Despite some turbulence in our lives, on the whole I'm glad we left when we did.

In the waiting area, noisy prostates are chatting and laughing, spurts of saliva in the air. I'm told I must provide a urine sample. Up 5 times in the night – but nothing now, so perverse is a mistreated bladder. I go into the swing-door toilet a few times to no end, then manage something. It's unacceptable.

On to the bier, immobilised, immediately I know I can produce whatever they want.

A new regime requires new tattoos. I'm marked up where the beam should cut along the flesh. Then the coccyx is dug into the hard black surface, giving the sort of pain that wipes out fear of death or incontinence.

I thought LA8 was supposed to be having a service. But no, here I am as usual. Yet perhaps it protests: something is wrong. It sings only one note not 3, and the furry red light stays on. Then red becomes green. I wait, tailbone squashed and arms in mummy-death pose, in case the red returns. Time has slowed. When the light is red again, LA8 manages 2 more notes. Surely it's out of order? I wait. Around go sun and moon, but the square eye doesn't travel right down, so that the moon box comes over my eyes.

I'm disorientated. I try positive thinking, a little self-love, but fail. Just as the tailbone is about to dissolve into gum, the girls come in.

I remark that the machine has been uncooperative. 'No,' they say, 'we took pictures.' In any case, it's not always the same treatment.

I'm polite and thank. But I suspect.

*

On television when people go into radiation zones they pad themselves out like moonwalking toddlers.

What if LA8 really did refuse to go forward and continued singing its notes into me, and I burst into internal flames, would they still say this was planned by the IT programme?

Is it the computer, the boffins, the girls, cool Dr Y, all thinking to control the machine? But here in this room it's just the 2 of us.

Willows whiten, aspens quiver by the shores of Gitche Gumee, says my brain. No, my addled mind; brains don't talk. Guide me O, O guide me. Pilgrim through this barren land.

I arrive home to be alerted by a son of Father's neighbour that he's not in his flat. I ring him. I visualise him lying on the floor in a mess of . . . I don't go there. That's the thing: no dignity and grace for us even in collapse, no pool of shiny ketchup. In the event, he isn't in a pool of anything. When I do reach him on his landline, he says he walked outside the door for a little fresh air, then returned just in case. I tell him to take his mobile phone when he goes out; that's why we got it for him. He says he does. I say, 'But you need to switch it on.' 'Ah yes,' he says, 'I must do that.'

I dash from the phone to the lavatory, then to the computer. I discover the children's writer Diana Wynn Jones survived cancer for nearly 2 years, but abandoned radiotherapy because of too much pain. I'm about to search for others who gave up when I'm called to the cubicle again. I need an iPad, then I could do 2 things together. The iPad could sit on the floor on the unsold copies, so I could read it when doubled up.

This is my second to worst day. Late in the afternoon a student comes to give me reiki – 'you don't have to believe,' she says. But there are many alternatives to chemical and mechanical treatments. She jolts me by asking if I thought it – the radiotherapy – was worth it, so grey I look.

You mean, just die now?

Nothing heroic about continuing, no failure in dying – or stopping.

'No,' I reply, 'I think I'll go on for a while.'

With Virginia Woolf's Mrs Dalloway: 'What she liked was simply life. "That's what I did it for," she said, speaking aloud to life . . .'

Or does the sympathetic student mean I grumble too much? Isn't your life extremely flat/With nothing whatever to grumble at?

Back on the laptop in the evening. I find Lorraine Day, who claims she refused radio and chemo, instead using the natural, simple, inexpensive therapies designed by God and outlined in the Bible. (God should know the antidote being the inventor of the problem.) She's not forthcoming about exactly what to eat and do – you have to buy the book or DVD for that. On the website a picture of the most enormous red tumour – it puts to shame Stage 1 – 3 clusters. Apparently it grew and grew before her very eyes, so that in 3 weeks it was almost an organ on its own. What can happen in 6 months, eh?

Then there's David Servan-Schriber: with his number-one bestselling cancer book. Apart from yoga, given up forever with the Lycra bottoms, and meditation, which failed to quiet the skittish 'monkey mind', the panacea is cruciferous vegetables. Cruciferae waving crosses as they march through guts. Wikipedia says these include cauliflower, cabbage, cress, bok choy, broccoli and similar green leaf plants. The very things forbidden for me by the Hospital Diet. Should I try them? Would they have rescued me from the Machine if ingested earlier and often?

We didn't eat a lot of leafy things when I was a child in hot places. Mother thought typhoid lurked in them; a friend of hers died from eating water-cress in Wales.

Beatrix Potter's Jeremy Fisher, a courteous frog, gave a dinner party of roast grasshopper with ladybird sauce for Sir Isaac Newton;

the other guest, Alderman Ptolemy Tortoise, brought his own salad in a string bag.

It's a fact: tortoises live longer than newts.

By chance yesterday in the long night I found a lump in one breast. I really wasn't looking. A mammogram is arranged for a week after radiotherapy. I will sit in the breast waiting-room – carpeted and better decorated because there's more money in breasts than pelvises, more feminine, though men too apparently. I shall watch anxious couples holding hands and panicking. I shall be smug. A breast can be hacked off. Whole books written about breasts. They even have a special saint – St Agatha holding her breasts like fried eggs on a platter.

No little pink bows and teddy bears for pelvics. No saint either. Am I feeling organ jealousy? Does breast cancer take on a little of that ennobling mythology of consumption?

While we pelvics stay embarrassed by our shameful predicament?

And yet. Let's all hold hands in the dark, breasts and pelvises and prostates.

17 January, Tuesday

The early morning news is full of the upturned *Costa Concordia*. So very tragic, yet so sadly on the edge of being not quite – or does my situation give dreadful things a ludic tinge? Those heart-rending little clumps of passengers waiting patiently in life jackets for rescue, while the junketing captain and crew sped off in a lifeboat. Pathos is stronger than tragedy, it makes you cry, it wraps round all tender, helpless things, little vulnerable furry creatures, rabbits and voles, made only to feed the fanged. All tear-jerking and almost funny.

*

2 Irishmen are talking loudly about prostates. I'm told I'll be on the machine not now but later, so I can see a doctor afterwards. Why am I out of my schedule? The girls fear the targeting has become imprecise.

'Imprecise!'

Where have rays been going all this time? Into the poor bladder again? Did the girls nod or view pictures of boyfriends or babies on their smart phones at the crucial moment? Did they let the machine wander off where it would, haphazardly burning?

A probe is inserted. Where exactly? I'm tied up gently with tapes by K. She asks if it's hurting. It isn't but the coccyx is moaning loudly as usual. A squashed back isn't a life-and-death matter. The coccyx – so far – doesn't leak, so we none of us care much about it. I keep silent.

At home I email PRADA. No reply.

I'm about to go on the Web in search of cancer drama when something troubles me. With or without Google, seeing what's in front of my nose or what's behind my myopic eyes, I feel the egoism and blandishments of illness.

What am I doing trying to equal Father who's so much further along the road, in so much more pain? As he was such a small part of my childhood, I wonder at my romanticising and containing of his larger-than-life self.

I recall my teen-age snippets: the end of Joyce's *Portrait of the Artist as a Young Man*, a diary entry by the callow hero, whom, at 16, I much admired. It's an 'epiphany', less Wordsworth's sudden awareness, more grandiloquent betrayal of something otherwise concealed: that anxiety about the father being there and not there, the son not giving enough and too much, being overwhelmed – or alienated – by his old stories. The son's boastful, egoistic posturing results in his writing the father over and over: 'I go to encounter for the millionth time the reality of experience and to forge in the smithy of my soul the uncreated conscience of my race.' (How male, I'd have said, if I'd met Joyce again at 30.) Then the end (my best snippet): 'Old father, old artificer, stand me now and ever in good stead.'

Cancer has stolen ecclesiastical terms: 'remission', 'recurrence', 'relapse', and my 'malignant' neoplasm. Why not filch 'epiphany': an unfettered moment when truth and error fuse?

Remember, medicine doesn't do irony.

18 January, Wednesday

No sunrise today, just black-grey dawn. Light rain makes everything look dirty and dim. But it's milder. Unpleasant murky promise of spring. Mid-winter's better, cleaner, clearer. You know where you are with it.

Christopher Smart wrote: 'there was no rain in Paradise because of the delicate construction of the spiritual herbs and flowers.' Dream of a drizzle-soaked Cambridge man.

Last night a friend said again to D, 'Is it really worth it? Does she really want to go on?' He repeats this to me. Sometimes people say, 'Surely there's a time to let go.'

Should I jauntily respond, 'Got to die some day'?

Neither D nor I think this a good idea.

Poor old bladder and bowels, I can't forsake you, though heaven knows you do misbehave. I know, I know it's the fault of the womb and its appendages. But still, you needn't have colluded like this. Well, you're getting your comeuppance.

A crowd of people are assembled by 7.45. Beginners ignorant of the ropes and ritual. LA8 has too many clients. I'm shunted to LA1.

A young man says he's off to put on the music. Please no, I say. But it bellows forth. I'm enveloped in a rhythm of Baby Baby

Something. Lilies whiten, aspens quiver again and again as I assert Eternal Providence to Justify all this.

At home I learn that a good friend, distinguished head of a cancer research unit in America, is losing her memory. Her amazing journey from rainy working-class Wigan to affluent sun-drenched California disappearing. I'm diminished every time a friend dies or loses what we shared. We used to speak, only sometimes, of that mixed relief and nostalgia felt when we thought of Wigan and Wales beside her oval pool under the palm trees. *Hiraeth*, I said. No such word in English.

When the time came, she and her husband planned to hire a plane and fly out to sea as far as petrol would take them. But she's left prematurely.

Very few very old people die in full possession of their faculties I read: all have dementia but some brains compensate – Father still doing intricate calculations near 100, though repeating stories. Why can't other organs behave so robustly and make up for weaker bits?

And yet, and yet, would we old be young if we could? Take away aches and pains and approaching death, and the answer may be, just may be, No. In old age you can see a life, really see it – well more of it. Before this, I think I liked being old. All passion spent? Maybe not quite, but obsessions much reduced. Contemplating, at the very best moments, a dignified, accepting farewell.

My life's been lived too early. 20, 30, 40 years on, everything will be so much better in or out of Hospital-land. There'll be gene therapy for cancer: busy curative cells rummaging around the body to root out bad ones. Or, after a life eating modified rice or barley to prevent degeneration, the wrong cholesterol and harmful memories, good cells and vibes will stay clear as day. If not, all troubles will be pharmaceuticalled away, no one will have to pull up socks ever again or get a grip of weak-willed organs on a hard bier.

The savage radiation machine will be placed in a museum to be stared at in wonder, along with leeches and tubes of mercury powder. (Yet I know that, if radiation could claim to cure asthma, I'd be back gazing at the beam. But I remember: at the outset of treatment, Dr Y announced there could be no more burning after this. NHS rationing or my enfeebled body?)

The green laser is aligned to my new tattoo marks. The flesh is prodded and pulled into place.

It's too late to find a cancer mantra for serenity, but at least the Shores of Gitche Gumee recede today. The quivering aspens are there though, and calm of mind, Tennyson's King Arthur always answering from his barge, never quite launching himself, the saddest man in literature. 'I have lived my life,' he keeps saying. I haven't quite, not even Under Milk Wood. I haven't properly seen dust in the air and 'children in the apple tree' either.

Let this be enough. No chemo please, no more cutting and scooping out. A long way to calm of mind, all passion spent. Kübler-Ross's people who accept death are just dead tired.

19 January, Thursday

Do I detect a slightly brighter morning? Warmth and light. Is this apricity – 'The warmeness of the Sunne in Winter'? Is the world turning?

Today I overhear – can you avoid it? – the matey, noisy whistling man planning to go to America for a golfing holiday when his (short) course is over. His cheeriness does us good, his whistling less. Behind him his diminutive wife scuttles unsmiling. The breast doesn't care for the whistling, but she's polite and keeps her eyes on her fashion magazine. (I still don't know why she's down here with us.) We've both avoided the stained seat. Her post-chemo hair is growing back thickly.

LA8 is having problems again. The sign on the notice board announces delays. I take out *White Fang*. I'm getting towards the end: it's turned into a sort of adult Beatrix Potter tale. Social Darwinism or the plasticity of clay, something like that. Hospital-land resembles *Peter Rabbit* and *White Fang*: underneath the girls' genuine, impersonal kindness, the decorous paper products and swing-door toilets, the business is violence. Not sexy, brutal, and voyeuristic; but shabby, 'for your own good'.

How wise to call the place Emmeline not Millicent; Pankhurst not Fawcett, violent suffragette not persuasive suffragist. You don't come here if you believe change can be brought about by good living and hope.

Since we expect to wait and wait until the dilatory machine shapes up, D wanders off to buy coffees for us both, small black decaf for me and perhaps something sugary and soft – I haven't managed any breakfast. Before he returns, LA8 pulls up socks and is ready to perform.

I'm urged on to the block against my protesting tailbone, so sore and raw now despite the sensitive cream I lather on it. I clench my fists against the pain and realise I'm starting arthritis in the right hand. Or is this the beginning of a splintering irradiated skeleton?

Poor old hands, already a geography of mountains and purple ridges. A young person's hand is almost a different genre, shining from within, no character in its blandness. But blandness is Beauty.

It takes longer than usual to stretch the flesh into proper alignment. I'm growing flabby and less taut with all this fibreless Victoria sponge; bones stick out like twigs. The placing has gone wrong. Tomorrow and tomorrow and tomorrow. Such a petty pace. 'If it were done when 'tis done,' twere well it were done quickly . . .' Never a truer thought, Will.

*

In the afternoon we fetch Father over for tea with a German couple. Usually so dapper and spruce, he looks shabby despite the jacket and tie. The 100 years pressing on him? More likely the bowels. Our secret.

I can't quite hear what he's saying, but it's something about mending his intricate carriage clock with a paperclip. My friends are a little bored. I'm hurt for him and exasperated by them and him. We're all too tired.

I hear my name and know my life's been taken into his narratives. On the whole his tales are cheerier than mine. Finding a rare tricycle for me after the war, helping me ride a two-wheeled bike in Bermuda, things I'd forget but for his stories, though I do remember Mother saying the bike would go back if I didn't learn to ride by the next day. That worked better than Father's patient pushing. He makes my nomadic childhood of 13 changes of school sound good – for me it's just a subject of competition: anyone been to more? Anyone had a worse divorce? Anyone had more illnesses? Anyone on a fourth cancer? Anyone got an older parent with more tales or opinions, more endless curiosity about people and things?

Hearing him, I wonder, and not for the first time, why I went on in this peripatetic, inflated fashion after I left 'home', changing jobs, houses, flats, partners: the fatal feeling of constraint and boundaries coming over me whenever nearly settled, the need to escape as soon as tied or moved in, to get on the road with my baggage. To follow the harsh tracks leading away and over the hill.

In the height of her misery over her faithless lover Gilbert Imlay, Mary Wollstonecraft admitted to wanderlust born of a shifting childhood. That need to imagine better places and people, starting again where no one knows you. When she went to Scandinavia, she was disappointed in its inhabitants; yet, when its harsh winter stopped her going farther north with baby Fanny, she was frustrated: surely there was a place where people were 'uncontaminated with cunning and censure'. A utopian elsewhere.

Father even recalls my little friend in the Welsh Council School whom I'd quite forgotten. The one always sick over his grey shorts after swallowing compulsory milk. But Father doesn't know that when I returned to that school for a few months – again – the teacher Mr Jones asked where I came from 'this time'. I said Bermuda. A crude canvas map of the world, much coloured imperial red, was rolled down the blackboard without a dot marking the tiny islands. Mr Jones grew irritable as the class tittered. 'Point to it, girl,' he said fingering his whipping bat, 'don't you know where you came from?' I stared at the map. Then he stabbed at Burma. 'There, girl, I'll do it for you. Did you ride an elephant?' I had to find a tongue and ride an elephant.

Which I did in Ceylon later, but not then.

After that I made up a good few tales as I moved from school to school. Especially in Dotheboys Hall. Why not? I was there because I'd answered on books I'd read only as Classic Comics. I wonder now why I invented Lithuanian parents with acres of potato fields – potatoes? – and Tamil writing – covering page after page of squiggles from right to left. One or 2 girls watched and believed. (Later, in my educated excitement at learning to condemn the British imperial adventure, I asked my elderly mother why she hadn't studied Tamil in Ceylon, instead of playing mah-jong with other European wives. 'People didn't,' she said. I squirm now for us both.)

I also told the girls about the great scaly lizards living underneath our house on Plantain Point, but nobody believed this, though it was true. It all passed the terrible time.

Years later my ordinary parents turned up. They'd travelled on a luxury liner – with Toby, the black-and-white-check tortoise, to which they'd secretly fed lettuce the whole way from Colombo to Southampton. 'One of us always ordered salad for lunch,' Mother said.

He survived the trip but couldn't adapt to the cold and, when we moved – again – to Scotland, began to hibernate. We tried him in the oven on a low setting. In the end we gave him, no questions asked, to the zoo in Edinburgh.

I left school before anyone could meet my parents. Probably nobody would have remembered their Lithuanian past.

In truth, they felt rather foreign to me.

Much, much later I met the headmistress and said how miserable I'd been. Why couldn't I have had the coconut Father thought it such a wheeze to dispatch with an address painted in black on its husk or the green rubber hot-water bottle Aunty sent to unfreeze my feet?

'You'd have been a malcontent anywhere,' she said, smiling out of her reptilian face.

Not so. If Ceylon wasn't the Garden of Eden, it was the next best thing. When ejected from Paradise, Adam landed in Ceylon and left his footprint on Adam's Peak. I've seen it. Perhaps Eve's was too delicate to leave a trace.

Yet something from the scenery round Dotheboys Hall got under my skin. Aching beauty arrives with puberty, and the volatile, jumping streams and swirling mist on moors will always be my scenic standard. Mostly there was gloom over the great mountain above the school but, when it suddenly emerged snow-covered before a blue sky, it was a marvel.

Father glossed the harshness of Wales as 'bracing': do other languages have such a word with its mix of virtue, exhilaration and threat?

I look over at him now on the sofa, my eyes closing with tiredness. My heart yearns for him. He's so old and works so hard not to feel unwanted. We want him. Very much. He's outlived his age and doesn't know how to tune his talk to just any listener. But he's all sympathy and generosity to anyone in need, to a young woman struggling up steps with a pushchair – happy now he's so ancient there's no offence in tickling an unknown baby – to the cleaning lady's wayward son, to the woman in the corner shop losing business to a new supermarket, to all people trying and striving, or sitting alone and sad on a park bench. Almost anyone down on luck or energy. As long as it's no taxman or union leader or woman 'who knows it all'.

More worldly-wise and shrewd, Mother used to try to rein in his generosity. Ceylon, for example.

They were motoring back to me – left home in a way social services would now rebuke. Driving down a straight, eye-closingly hot jungle road, Father ploughed the Austin A40 into a stout buffalo. Amazingly, the buffalo was wounded but not killed, while the car was demolished and my parents, bruised and shaken, needed stitches from the local doctor. Over the next months, the owner of the buffalo cycled to our house declaring his livelihood impaired by the wounding of his beast. Father paid up; Mother warned of escalation. True enough: the owner's brother appeared, then the second brother, then cousins, then a group of children from the second brother. Father continued to pay out, making (of course) a humorous story of it all.

So, too, the cook's brother's wedding. We'd the only electricity out on the Point and the cook asked for a link to it, so as to allow a light on the event beyond flares and a kerosene lamp. We'd gone round the harbour to a get-together organised by parents of my friend Pat. Looking out through the dark, one of the guests feared a fire at our place since the promontory, usually almost pitch black at night, was glowing. As we rushed back I was anxious for the chipmunk which I put to bed each night in his cage and my Classic Comics. Toby would weather a fire and jackal-dogs know what to do. Approaching the house, we found the fire clarifying into a fairground. Fairy lights in all colours looped across palm trees, then trailed down to the water. It was so spectacular that Father was almost elated until, at Mother's bidding, he went to turn the electricity off and found the metre hand going round so fast the dial was too hot to touch. The light, dancing and smell of spiced food were so joyous and the cook and guests so loudly grateful that Father hadn't the heart to end it all. 'Till midnight,' he said, and the whole party cheered him. 'Such a soft touch,' said Mother.

Father loved the mathematics of money and finance but had no care for saving unless to give away.

20 January, Friday

LA8 is resting and I'm on LA1. I'm prodded on to the bier by unfamiliar hands. For a moment the pain is piercing. They mean well, as Mother often remarked when people were especially beastly.

After all these weeks I notice for the first time that the ceiling above LA1 has circles inside the square panels where LA8's room has only squares, like the map of an American city. The circles look a little cleaner, newer. Have I given my loyalty to the wrong machine? Is LA8 my 'love god', like Jack London's white-man owner of White Fang? Will I finish this ridiculous novel by the time it's all over? If I have 5 months of chemo what will I read then? I did Book I of Proust after the hysterectomy for cancer 2, trying to overcome my (sexist) desire for a female nurse to stop my messy crawling to the bathroom.

Back on the chairs with the breast lady, I await my last review. She says she's in a research trial group and has confidence she'll not be ill again. I smile back.

Jung says cancer is symbolic. But, as Bolingbroke remarked to old father Gaunt, who can cloy the hungry edge of appetite by bare imagination of a feast? Tell me that, Carl? I've thought a lot about hale organs but produce no smooth results.

Jung had a patient, a brilliant scientist – always 'brilliant' in anecdotes – without emotional ties or religion, who suddenly believed he had a stomach cancer. This cancer didn't exist although he suffered its terrors. But he was a masculine chap, a scientist, and could only lose his anxiety and his imaginary cancer by reintegrating his feminine spiritual side into his psyche.

Perhaps my feminine side needs attention. My cake-making is poor. I must elbow D out of the kitchen and make a Victoria sponge, then offer it, not eat it. But no, I am on no universal journey. It's Real Cancer and whose fault is it? Surely not mine?

Another worrying pastoral review intended to comfort. The mean statistics can't be made to lie. Why not? Politicians do. I do.

I go home and walk very slowly to the Library close by, to get more books on death. As soon as I mount the steps, I know I'm in a bubble. Will the bubble pop, will I leak from the bowels or bladder or head? Which orifice will let me down? Am I radioactive, or radiopassive, moonlike or sunlike? If the lights were dim would I shine – all of me or just the bladder or bowels or what's left of the genitals, glowing luminous like the X-rays at Security – the pitiful inside of a suitcase faulted for too many millilitres of cheap eau de Cologne?

I must go home. I'm not fit to read books or order them up. Bowels used to be the seat of emotions, better than the heart, but they were further up then, somewhere nearer the lungs.

I go back down the Library steps, counting. It's drizzling. I then count paces along the road. *Un, dau, tri, pedwar, pump* . . . Why in Welsh? I haven't lived in Wales this half century and more. What's it doing here in this flat, damp town?

After a few sessions in my cubicle, I lie on the bed. I must be positive, appreciate what I have. At last I ring the friendly lady from Bury.

She's contacted the hospital twice to give me her phone number and I'm remiss. Her car tends now to go unaided to the hospital, she says. Her husband has an infection and can't yet eat ordinary food. She gives him just a little porridge. I love the idea of this caring for another. It makes me feel teary.

I think of D. I will never tell him how the Victoria sponge starts to stick where it shouldn't.

23 January, Monday

The very last week of the machine. The wind whistles through me, I'm a china eggcup, a lacuna, an aporia. Nothing between stomach and pan. Is there Cancer Anonymous? Can I stand up and declare, My name is JT and I am Cancerous.

I dash to the lavatory through the night. By morning just malodorous liquid. Joyce's Bloom took pleasure in the rising smell of his defecated breakfast kidneys. Can't emulate this.

By now the sky is whitening when D and I reach the hospital. Regulars arrive, some exchange greetings. I feel irritable. I don't like people indulging in pleasantries. I want them to sit in silence. I'm like Mr Glowry in Peacock's *Nightmare Abbey*, the 'atrabilarious' patriarch who demands all round him echo his melancholy by showing 'a long face or a dismal name'. (Actually both: he fires a Diggory Deathshead, who turns out to be cheerful.)

Today there's an interchange between 2 new breasts about hair growth after chemo – does it come through grey or dark, curly or straight? – and about reconstruction or not. Wives of prostates join in. One says her husband can't remember when to take his chemo pills even when it's on his smart phone; she should put it on his forehead so he'd see it when he looked in the mirror.

Everyone laughs after each remark. Except me. I am glum. I spend time in the lavatory hitching up my unshapely red skirt. When I come out the breasts are gone. Were they in the wrong place?

In the machine room I ask about the more repulsive of my present symptoms. They are usual, all quite usual. Machines are indiscriminate in what they attack and the poor organs quiver and tremble and try to withstand the onslaught. What can they do but spit and eject? It's their way.

I no longer feel close to LA8 — -it sings as ever, but the girls are not the original ones and my routine has changed for these final sessions. The machine doesn't travel behind as it used to and its growling purr is longer, its song less distinct. The coccyx is still almost numb with pain.

Che sara sara goes round and round. Some enchanted evening, a long long way to Tipperary, now the day is over, night is drawing nigh, shadows of the evening steal across the sky.

I mean to read Kübler-Ross properly, not just look up the stages. The book is prefaced by the prayer of St Francis which Mrs Thatcher so hilariously quoted at the beginning of her agitating reign.

Death is a subject that's evaded, ignored, and denied by our youth-worshipping, progress-oriented society, says K-B. So? Why not? It's an end, and who spends time on ends?

I Google her to see what she knew and find she made it to 78. A little longer than I've had. But paralyzed for nearly a decade, so ready for death. Think about your own death, she says, it's part of human growth. Like cancer? Death is not an enemy to be conquered. Live fully the years you have, however short. You only know the shortness when too late. Death is a friendly companion on life's journey.

Live each day 'as 'twere your last', we sang in school assembly. Steve Jobs said, 'If you live each day as if it was your last, some day you'll most certainly be right.'

D and I go to Father's flat. On his desk he has early daffodils with frilly trumpets in a blue vase from the patrons of the pub he fears now to visit. Such charming people, he says. Always so kind. He's in obvious pain but doesn't want to show it, especially before D. I tell him that in hospital I remembered the journey from Ceylon with Mother, which I hadn't thought of in years. Journeys are longer when you're a child he says and tells me again his own epic one. I know it as if it were mine: I look at him but hardly listen.

His gassed father dead, the family of the great house bankrupt and the pretty thatched tied cottage no longer theirs, mother and 4 little children walking along the road behind a cart holding all their possessions. Distant kin sorry for their plight, so each taking in a boy. Father leaving his home of rook pies, haystacks, bee hives and hunted rabbits for an industrial Midland city of blackened back-to-back houses: such horror. What was a boy to do but one day walk away from it all and go west to green fields and a mother who was always and would always be there?

Sometimes he's 9 when this happens, sometimes 10, a stocky child with light brown hair and eager eyes. Mostly she walks to meet him when she's heard he's coming, but sometimes he travels alone, a plucky, courteous boy knowing what he wants.

24 January, Tuesday

The penultimate day. I fear flatness, the undramatic vacuous after-wards. Much as I so want it to end.

On LA8. Without M or any of the usual girls, it seems a more alien machine. But the song is the old one, and the frying part happens each time on the side thrusts. This is the boost to the 'vaginal vault' mentioned on my amended schedule. The cathedral I've become, with its hollow alabaster tomb below.

On the slab I find I'm feeling neutral towards Consultant X. Have I reached Kübler-Ross's acceptance?

Unlikely. It simply needs more energy to blame than I can muster. I've had a lobotomy by proxy: with slash and burn below, the head received the bigger blow.

I oughtn't to go on working. I know, I know. My colleagues must look askance. How can they be strategic in their thinking, how line-manage, think blue-skies and major fund-raising campaigns, with me like a cat tangling their straightened skeins?

I do appreciate your tolerance very much. When I first moved into the roomy college house – with cancer 1, trying so hard to hide the fact – I ended twice in A&E: none of you mentioned the ambulance whining up the gravel driveway.

In my long wheezing attic nights while rain drubbed on the Welsh slates, Mother read Jonathan Bing to me. Invited to take tea with the King, he tries to go but something is always wrong, he's never in the right place, never has the right words, never wears the right clothes – he sports pyjamas on his last attempt. Finally, he goes home and writes a note to the King, 'If you please will excuse me, I won't come to tea; for home's the best place for all people like me.'

But where's home? Mole had his hole, Jeremy Fisher his damp house. Working was always my hole, not a place on a map at all. I want to go on 'working'. Nowhere else to be.

Then to Father by myself. He's lonely in his small flat, going nowhere, not even to his beloved park, for fear, big fear, and rightly. Swallowing packets of antibiotics through his sandpapered throat, series after series, and almost nothing else. He's becoming a bag of bones. Neither I nor the Baby caught *C.difficile* – it propagates only in Hospital-land, just as I read – but on poor Father it's taken stern hold.

Why will no one help him?

'I shouldn't have been sent out so soon,' he says again and again. I know, I know, but what can we do? He rings the GP, I ring the GP, but it's catch as catch can to get them in their flexi-time, and another hurdle, never to be jumped, to attract the attention of Miss G away in Hospital-land. (Why can't we have access to our own records — would this be revolution?)

'I'm wearing out,' he says, 'my body's shutting down. I've had a good innings.' He loves cricket and its metaphors, its sticky wickets, its stumps, good openers and straight bats.

'But not before the 100th birthday, you can't.' Remember, you'll be 100, the Baby one. That's Something. And what about the Royal Telegram? 'You've never given up before.'

'No,' he says sadly, 'I haven't given up.'

A friend from the pub has just brought him an orchid with entrancing spotted petals. He points this out. I too have an orchid from a kind student. But I don't look at it as he looks at this one. He loves flowers, planted in parks and wild in country hedgerows. He knows all their names. Nobody relishes the spring park as he does. His pleasure is worth all the Council spends on regimented beds.

I shouldn't, he shouldn't, we shouldn't, we say. We're moral generations but not now of consequence.

He's carefully dressed in his jacket and neatly tied tie; the ironed white handkerchief shows above his breast pocket. His shabby neatness emphasises his frailty, his new thinness. I too have lost weight despite the Victoria sponge and sticky toffee puddings, just old muscle made new flab. But I'm nothing to this dwindling, this wasting.

Could he be turning his face to the wall like Aunty and Myfanwy? But that's Mother's folk, not his; he's from sturdier stock. But none so old as this.

Perhaps, after all, it's the end. Let the darkness come, I hope I don't say. Please no. He will never whisper, 'Time to let go.' He can't and shouldn't.

Wearing out is one thing – giving up quite another.

I see he's staring with his one blurry eye, out of features both gaunt and sagging, at the back of an old Christmas card envelope.

He's scribbling something with real ink. Figures.

He says, 'Between us I think we should manage to buy one of these new ISAs for the Baby.'

25 January, Wednesday

Before the Shipping Forecast, I begin to think of the Future. I'd resolved against this – but fresh woods and pastures new, however much shores and sounding seas wash away a friend's corpse. Milton couldn't help it in *Lycidas*. No more can I. Not a matter of letting the darkness come or disappear, no will involved. Just sneaks up.

Who'll say there's as much happiness on this globe as it's 'capable of affording'? asked Mary Wollstonecraft in one of her rare upbeat moods.

The final appointment to hear the results is 2 months away or, with my luck, more like 3, even 4. There'll be CT and MRI scans and on my part much speculation. Will the errant cells still be procreating after this blasting? How could they? The sluts.

At last Jane Austen comes in handy: receiving beloved Wentworth's letter, Anne Elliot realises all the world could do for her depends on its contents. The world hasn't done a lot for me recently. It owes me. This will be its moment to pay up.

I won't anticipate, I will not. Then I begin.

To prepare for the worst?

You're never prepared for the very very worst, for the worst is unimaginable. *Et in arcadia ego*, and not only in Arcadia. The longest journey isn't marriage, Shelley, it's the time between fearing and knowing.

What news does it bring – good or bad? the impatient ask in *Pride and Prejudice*. 'What is there of good to be expected?' replies Mr Bennet.

K, the radiologist, will be present and look with compassionate eyes upon me. But I won't need compassion, for I'll be almost detached after a long wait in the corridor, stomach-churning quite past. That's the purpose. Humpty Dumpty sat for ever on a wall, only then had his great fall.

Young Dr Y will give the faintest smile as she swishes back her smart black bob. Not a people person but a straight one. She doesn't waste words. We have back your results, she'll say and use my first name – or will she be less familiar because the case is serious? No matter, we have your results, she'll say smiling or unsmiling, and I won't ask too quickly: it's good for patients to show restraint.

The radiotherapy will have worked or not worked – I do the second scenario.

There's a reasonable chance that it's failed. If it has, the only way forward will be drastic mutilation. We can cut you open and try to remove the vigorous cancer cells from your now scant body. We can dig them out, though in the process you'll lose bits you'd rather retain – bladder, bowels, kidneys, that kind of offal. Those poor things have taken such a bruising. That is, if we don't think you Too Old for Treatment.

Old people always clamour for an operation.

I'll nod, because I'm my head now. There isn't much left inside, so losing a little more will be neither here nor there.

Bags to dangle afterwards for the various wastes that need to exit. Plenty of people have them. You don't always know.

The owners do though.

Or she could do a Consultant X and tell me I'll be fine and keep the rest to herself.

By the way — and I've checked on this with the Macmillan booklets — the bowel and bladder and intestinal side-effects you now have are permanent. Dr Y will point this out.

I end the home movie. Hitching up my baggy skirt, I set off with D for my final appointment with the machine. I dash into the lavatory on the way from the car park down the corridors of bicycle poem and mountain pictures. When we arrive in the waiting area, the laughing prostate and his wife are there, but he's not laughing today. The whistling man is late but I hear him in the distance coming towards us.

I sit tensed up as far as I can, orifices as tight as tight can be. Avoid the wind: you don't know where it leads. All down there so secretive. Unseemly, indecorous — but it's what we irradiated think about, night and day. Those of us who've stayed the course.

Shouldn't we congratulate ourselves just a little? We haven't faltered. Indeed, we've been quite upset if interrupted, when Christmas interfered and New Year, which we'd no wish to celebrate.

But, from now on, I'll be alone: no pleasant girls to mention the unmentionable to, no one to ask even summarily about my functions. So often I've resolved to formulate a gracious response to routine queries. How will I stop telling people who expect 'Fine' and 'Well' that, 'No, I am not fine', that I have had since waking 6 sessions of . . . How respond to the startled look and stop long before I achieve disgust with my failed inhibitions. How remember that I'm outside, not *in* Hospital-land?

For my last session, I'm on LA1. An unsentimental place of brisk detachment. Perhaps it's as well I can't make a play of thanks to either LA8 or its servers.

I stare at the circles on the ceiling for the last time, and the machine gives its final song, faster than usual, with elongated sounds only on the right side of me.

I ask if the new sound means anything?

Do they know what's happened? Has all this worked? Been working? Has It Been Worth It?

The photos say 'Nothing'.

Oh, I know that, I only ask.

Come on, make that 'Nothing' heroic. It's a good word. Far more than the 'Something' that so dazzled cunning Lizzie Bennet when she thought of being Mistress of Pemberley.

By the shop door in her claustrophobic village, Emma sees 'nothing that does not answer', not even curs quarrelling over a dirty bone. At the close of life, Jane A wanted 'nothing but death'. (Fame too no doubt, but not just then). The Sibyl of Cumae said much the same when reduced to dust in a jar for forgetting to ask Apollo for healthy youth as well as longevity.

On Margate Sands.
I can connect
Nothing with nothing.

The pain has been real and is real – but am I also suffering, just a little, from melodrama in the Waste Land of Hospital-land; Dr Google in cahoots with my valetudinarian self?

Have I walked into the lodging-house in Sanditon and sat down with Jane Austen's energetic Parkers in a comedy of illness, a 'supererogatory wretchedness'?

I do hope so.

Much worse and far longer ordeals out there. I'm well aware. Take Father – and almost all the dead.

I exit into the waiting area like any other day and see the panda-eyed woman in the poncho (so she hadn't escaped after all) and a new prostate couple with worn faces and high cheekbones: morose, resigned like the pair in *American Gothic*. I catch the woman's tired, unblinking eye but neither of us smiles. I sit down to wait for a leaflet about After-effects and Long-term pelvic problems.

I open up *White Fang*, and find that, with no planning, I'm on the last tear-jerking page. It jerks no tear from me.

The nurse who gives me the booklets says that the present exaggerated side-effects will carry on undiminished for 10 days or so. 'Stay with the white bread and sponge cake for 2 or 3 months,' she advises, perhaps longer. 'Add other foods slowly.'

I don't look at D, whose cookery-books of fancy olive breads and bean and lentil curries have been unopened for so long. Make a record of what you eat and what you . . .

Will this take the place of the daily machine and its ritual?

The receptionist smiles impersonally, says Good bye and Good luck. It's been a pleasant unit all told, not an easy job, pummelling and pushing our anxious bodies, serving temperamental machines in cold rooms, at the beck and call of sardonic green and red lights. I'm grateful.

I arrive home. I pack up my books on death and grieving and, after the morning sessions in the lavatory and before the afternoon fatigue sets in, hitch up my red skirt and set off to return them to the Library. I leave after placing them on the reception desk. No one asks details as I flee. Then D drives me to Father, so I needn't shuffle into McDonald's clean facilities.

He's had a terrible night and day with no respite or help. He's grey and wan. After a little bowel chitchat, he smiles and remarks, 'P says there are crocuses in the park already.'

'Hmm,' I say, not quite sharing his temperament, but liking the idea of crocuses.

Postscript

Why publish this diary? Why overcome revulsion at embarrassing afflictions? One reason is that a publisher has kindly wanted to publish it.

I feel some embarrassment at not being dead, but have overcome it. I must however prepare for deflating comments from my instinctively reticent generation: 'How brave of you.' 'I could never have . . .' Saying to a friend if not to me, 'Personally, I'd rather take my clothes off and dance naked along the high street.'

So why the compulsion to relate and reveal?

Perhaps it's useful to add my voice to sufferers who lament delays in treatment. Useful also to highlight the fact that radiotherapy, like cancer itself, damages the body forever, and urge doctors to do more for those they've nuked and left with the aftermath. But, in reality, I have no compelling answer beyond a common desire to declare I was here and this happened to me, that the words might stay a little longer than I usually fear *I* will. I could have avoided the murky details to shield myself and family, but where's the point in reticence when details are the story and my family's robust?

Memories and unaccustomed introspection have brought back a past not often scrutinised, but I can't say they've dented my ignorance of a self honed largely in solitude – though perhaps I've come to see my bumpy life (at intervals) as better than I usually say it was. Yet, though the present is good, barring sloppy health, I would still like to have had a different past – and temperament.

Ahead of treatment, I wish I'd known more of what would happen both in the process and in effects; perhaps if anyone facing radio-therapy reads this, it might point to some of what could be in store and be helpful, or cautionary.

If asked whether the treatment was worth it now it's over, I'd say, of course, definitely. If you have consciousness and words, anything's worth it. Maybe even without words, though I couldn't go that far myself.

As the girls said, no one wanted to be there, but, since I was, it was not – with hindsight – so bad a place to be. I have paid National Insurance for many decades, but, even if I hadn't, this treatment would have been free. For that, many thanks. The hiccups and failures on the way, especially for Father, were real – they could be avoided with better communication between GPs and hospitals, patients and consultants. We're not fools out here: we may not know technical terms, but we know feelings and fears.

I have the promised side-effects. They're unsocial and debilitating but not totally destructive. (As foretold, pelvic bones did grow weak and break on both sides – the college provided a wheelchair when needed and kind P. D. James, whom I last met when we talked over her Jane Austen sequel, brought round a contraption on 3 wheels to steady my steps. But now the wheelchair and contraption are returned and crutches put away in a cupboard. I'm precariously upright again and can walk in flat warm places, though there'll be no more tramping over strenuous hills. I was never expert at fighting off disease, am less so now, and, if cancer is for the moment at bay, asthma is not; but asthma and I are old bedfellows.) Slowly over the months I weaned myself off the austerity of sponge cake and boiled rice, then re-discovered the exuberant taste of garlic, chest-nuts and black beans. G & T too.

I find my mid-70s a good time to start over without overweening expectations, ambition having cooled from any agitating boil. (Now I'm here, I wish I hadn't waited for the intimacy with death to feel that cooling.) I write the novels I was too busy to write when I had to make a living for a family, taking demanding, better-paid jobs against inclination to keep us all going – when perhaps we might happily have managed on less. I won't win the Man-Booker prize or pen a best-selling or 'feel-good' tale, but writing without anxiety over protocol is fun. With it you can manipulate memories that simply swarm and settle when left to themselves. And invent different alternative and parallel lives. The days or years being short, this seems a pleasing use of them.

Montaigne again: 'There is nothing more notable in Socrates than that he found time, when he was an old man, to learn music and dancing, and thought it time well spent.'

I'll read and write as long as I can: there's nothing certain but uncertainty – and colds in winter.

Father lived to watch with delight the Baby crawl on the grass and wiggle a daisy. He shuffled into the park to gaze at crocuses, then daffodils, striped tulips, and red, orange and white roses, but not the dark-leaved dahlias he so admired. He was taken to hospital just before his 100th birthday. On the big day, a card from Iain Duncan Smith, Secretary of State for Work and Pensions, sat at the top of the pile. For a dreadful instant we feared the Queen had abrogated her royal duty. Then, halfway down, the monarch in full-face colour congratulated him on his achievement of years.

'Right,' said Father, and was pleased.

Pleased too when my friend H brought him a Cornetto ice cream and a nephew sent him *The Times* from August 1912. Its title page of births, deaths, detail of the '*Titanic* disaster' and a plea for money by an 'Orphan Infant Asylum' for children from the Empire. Had he had more time, he'd have spent it happily exclaiming over each yellowing column.

A few days on, Father was moved to the hospice. Then returned to hospital. We were summoned to his bedside. Knowing we were there for impending death, since a nurse brought in tea and *chocolate* biscuits. (Digestive biscuits follow anaesthetic or modest grief.) The Baby tottered around pulling at tubes, Father's one eye catching him whenever it could.

Something in the smell in the room set off boyhood memory and he spoke of keeping the smithy's fire going as horses were shoed with a red-hot iron.

Abruptly he stopped talking. His hands grew cold. We felt tears starting. Then, before we could quite take it in, the hands we held began to get warm and assume colour. He opened his eye and continued where he'd left off.

He was sent back to the hospice. On his last day, just after the Baby's first birthday, he asked if, in time, he could move into the bed on the other side of the room, where his one working eye would see the flowerbed.

He died too soon.

A Disclaimer

We children of the Second World War owe a huge debt to England's National Health Service: any criticism I've made here is in this context. I've described what I felt day-by-day during a session of radical radiotherapy: my panicky opinions, uninformed by medical knowledge, are 'the measure of my sight, not the measure of things', to quote Montaigne again.

When concluded, I found the diary had delivered fragments of auto-biography. More jointed memories arrived at less stressed and painful moments; the disjointed bubbled up during treatment.

I have no close relatives in my generation: so the story-of-self is unverified.

I've changed initials and identifying circumstances of everyone closely involved, beyond my immediate family.

Acknowledgments

I owe thanks to Derek Hughes for invaluable comments on the diaries, also to Pat Tate and Dan Mercola for most useful advice. My main gratitude is to Katherine Bright-Holmes for her generous help and encouragement.

A Selection of Janet Todd's Previous Works

Women's Friendship in Literature (New York: Columbia University Press, 1980, 1984, 1992)

English Congregational Hymns in the Eighteenth Century; their purpose and design (Watts to Cowper), co-authored with M. Marshall (Lexington: University of Kentucky Press, 1983)

Sensibility: An Introduction (London: Methuen, 1986)

Feminist Literary History (Cambridge: Polity Press; New York: Routledge, 1988)

The Sign of Angellica: Women, Writing and Fiction 1660 – 1800 (London: Virago, 1989; New York: Columbia University Press, 1990, 1992)

Gender, Art and Death (Cambridge: Polity Press, 1993)

The Critical Fortunes of Aphra Behn (London and New York: Boydell and Brewer, 1998)

The Revolutionary Life of Mary Wollstonecraft (London: Weidenfeld and Nicolson; New York: Columbia University Press, 2000; London: Bloomsbury eBook, 2013)

Rebel Daughters: Ireland in Conflict (London: Viking, 2003) *Daughters of Ireland: The Rebellious Kingsborough Sisters and the Making of a Modern Nation* (New York: Ballantine Books, 2004)

Cambridge Introduction to Jane Austen (Cambridge: Cambridge University Press, 2006)

Death and the Maidens: Fanny Wollstonecraft and the Shelley Circle (London: Profile Books; Berkeley: Counterpoint Press, 2007)

Jane Austen: Her Life, Her Times, Her Novels (London: André Deutsch, 2014, 2017)

Lady Susan Plays the Game (London: Bloomsbury, eBook 2013; paperback, 2016)

A Man of Genius (London: Bitter Lemon Press, 2016, 2017)

Aphra Behn: A Secret Life (London: Fentum Press, 2017)

Selected Editions since 1990

The Complete Works of Mary Wollstonecraft (7 vols, with Marilyn Butler; London: Pickering and Chatto, 1989; New York: New York University Press, 1990)

Wollstonecraft, Mary, *Mary, A Fiction and Maria*; Shelley, Mary, *Matilda* (London: Pickering and Chatto, 1991; London: Penguin, 1992)

Behn, Aphra, *Oroonoko, The Rover and Other Works* (London: Penguin, 1992)

The Complete Works of Aphra Behn (7 vols; London: Pickering & Chatto; Columbus: Ohio State University Press, 1992 – 6; London: Routledge ebook, 2018)

Love-Letters between a Nobleman and his Sister (London: Penguin, 1996)

The Political Writings of Mary Wollstonecraft (London: Pickering and Chatto; Toronto: University of Toronto Press, 1993; Oxford University Press, 1994)

Counterfeit Ladies: Mol Cutpurse and Mary Carleton (with Elizabeth Spearing) (London: Pickering and Chatto; New York: New York University Press, 1994)

The Complete Letters of Mary Wollstonecraft (London: Penguin, 2003; New York: Columbia University Press, 2004)

Aphra Behn's Oroonoko (London: Penguin, 2003)

The Cambridge Edition of the Works of Jane Austen (General Editor) (Cambridge: Cambridge University Press, 2005 – 08)

Joint editor (with Antje Blank) of *Persuasion* (2006); (with Linda Bree) of *Manuscript Works* (2008)

Selected Edited Collections

A Dictionary of British and American Women Writers, 1660 – 1800 (Lanham: Rowman and Littlefield, 1985)

Aphra Behn Studies (Cambridge: Cambridge University Press, 1996)

Cambridge Companion to Aphra Behn (with Derek Hughes) (Cambridge: Cambridge University Press, 2004)

Jane Austen in Context (Cambridge: Cambridge University Press, 2008)

Cambridge Companion to Pride and Prejudice (Cambridge: Cambridge University Press, 2013)